BEYOND THE HYPE

The Inside Story of Science's Biggest Media Controversies

HYPE

FIONA FOX

Elliott&Thompson

First published 2022 by
Elliott and Thompson Limited
2 John Street
London WC1N 2ES
www.eandtbooks.com

ISBN: 978-1-78396-617-2

9 8 7 6 5 4 3 2 1

A catalogue record for this book is available from
the British Library.

Typesetting by Marie Doherty
Printed by CPI Group (UK) Ltd,
Croydon, CR0 4YY

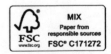

For Declan

and

*For Professor Sir Colin Blakemore, who personifies everything
I have come to hold dear in science: the excellence in his research;
the firm belief that engaging with the media is central to being
a great scientist; and the courage and bravery to defend science
under attack, way before there was the strength in numbers to
give him cover and support. The SMC is imbued with Colin's
values, and I am proud that we are one of his many legacies.*

'*You are doing better in the features pages and magazines of the broadsheets who are covering science more widely than ever before ... but this is not the case on the front-line of news reporting. BSE may have no link with CJD and hard-working scientists may have got us out of a terrible mess – but the public has yet to be convinced. One renegade doctor may have destroyed the MMR programme while best research shows that the vaccine is safe – but the public has yet to be convinced. GM foods may pose no proven risk and indeed may hold huge potential benefits for mankind – but the public has yet to be convinced. This is not down solely to the vagaries of an irresponsible press. It is also down to the failure of the majority of scientists to stand and be counted in the eyes of the public and put their case across convincingly.*'

Simon Pearson, night editor at *The Times* and
founding SMC board member, in a speech to
scientists at the Royal Society, 2002

CONTENTS

INTRODUCTION

'Cancer jab alert after girl dies', screamed the news headlines in September 2009 when fourteen-year-old schoolgirl Natalie Morton tragically died after receiving the human papillomavirus (HPV) vaccine at her school. The rollout of the cervical cancer vaccine programme in schools had already been controversial among some members of the public, particularly religious groups, who took issue with under-sixteens being vaccinated against a sexually transmitted virus. Now concerns about the vaccine's safety took centre stage and the story was headline news for several days. Ten years later I asked the audience at a science festival for a show of hands of those who remembered it, but there were none. When I asked who had heard of the row over whether the measles, mumps and rubella vaccine (MMR) causes autism – a row that first hit the headlines in 1998 – every hand in the audience went up.

Why did one vaccine scare story enter the public consciousness when another barely registered? My answer, and the theme of this book, is that scientists found their voice, in part because of an organisation that I set up. The Science Media Centre (SMC) was established in 2002. We have pioneered a new proactive approach to science in the headlines based on our founding philosophy that 'the media will do science better when scientists do the media better'. The easiest and best way to improve the media coverage of science is for scientists to work with journalists to help them get their stories right.

Today, the SMC has over three thousand leading scientists on our database, is used by every national news outlet in the UK, and runs around sixty press conferences a year. Funded by small donations from more than a hundred organisations, we have spawned a network of SMCs in countries around the world, including Australia, Canada, New Zealand and Germany, and an organisation doing some of what we do in the USA. Recent additions include Taiwan and a pan-continental organisation for Africa, with a new centre due to open in Spain in early 2022.

When the first journalist called us in 2009 about Natalie Morton's death, I contacted every vaccine expert on our database asking for instant reaction to the breaking news. Over the next hours and days, many of them did the rounds of TV newsrooms and their comments were quoted all over the press. Fact boxes, Q&As and clear graphics that they had helped to create appeared next to scary headlines about this awful and unexpected death. None of these scientists knew the precise details about the individual case of course, but that was no reason not to engage: instead, they talked about the mountain of data showing the safety and effectiveness of this vaccine. Within hours of the story breaking, the headlines started to change. 'Cancer jab is safe, say the experts', read the *Daily Mail*.

In the past scientists had tended to steer clear of the media, understandably preferring the laboratory to the glare of the spotlight. There was not yet a consensus on the importance of accessible science communication as a public good, and few incentives for academics to take part in any public engagement. Those who did so tended to be science popularisers with a flair for communicating their field of research or explaining the way that science works, but they were few and far between. But things were changing. In 1985 the Royal Society published a report called 'The Public Understanding of Science', also known as the Bodmer Report, calling on scientists to see public engagement as their public duty. By the late 1990s funders had started to introduce incentives for media work, including making grants conditional on researchers sharing their results with the public. These initiatives were having an impact: scientists had begun dipping their toes into media work, explaining their findings to trusted science journalists. But there was still a problem when controversial stories about science hit the headlines: researchers were much less used to wading into huge media rows that pitted them against campaigners or patient groups, and they were generally reluctant to engage. That exacerbated the media frenzy, allowing inaccuracies to flourish, with implications both for public understanding of science and public policy more widely.

But something new and significant had happened in the case of the HPV scare. Rather than run away from a difficult or sensationalised story with the potential to damage or discredit their work, scientists had run towards it. This was a tragic and terrible case but the wider reporting on it was accurate and informed as a result of their engagement, and this in turn led to a greater public understanding of the evidence on vaccines.

So what changed? I'd love to say it was all thanks to us. But to really understand the extent of the change in science, you first need to know why the SMC came to exist in the first place.

***

The row over the MMR vaccine wasn't the only science story to make the front pages at the turn of the new millennium: animal research facilities and the introduction of genetically modified (GM) foods, for example, were also attracting negative attention and misinformation. There were a few bold scientists willing to step into these stories but not enough to prevent the public and policy makers being misled.

Most scientists working in these fields actively avoided talking to the press, choosing to remain cocooned in their universities and research institutes, designing their next field trials, or preparing new findings for publication in peer-reviewed journals. Plant scientists in world-class research institutes told me how they watched, bewildered, as media-savvy campaigners from Greenpeace and Friends of the Earth joined forces with the tabloids to demonise and discredit the promise of GM technology. The result? The public, the politicians and the supermarkets all delivered a resounding 'no' before a single GM crop had even been developed.

In 1999 the ineffective response of the scientific community to such media furores became the focus of a House of Lords Select Committee on Science and Technology. The report of the Science and Society inquiry, brainchild of then science minister Lord Sainsbury and chaired by the late Lord Jenkin, is now studied in science communication courses as one of the seminal works on the public understanding of science. It is a fascinating reminder of the tense relationship between science and the media at the end of the last millennium: eminent scientists would bemoan the media coverage and accuse journalists of undermining public trust in science, while science journalists would point the finger firmly back at aloof and elitist scientists, blaming them for emerging once a year to deliver truth on tablets of stone and then retreating back into the safety of academia. Pallab Ghosh, science reporter at the BBC, urged scientists to stop whingeing about the rules of the game, roll up their sleeves and get on the pitch.

Published in February 2000, the final Science and Society report called for the investment of new resources to encourage and train more scientists to engage with the media. It concluded:

> The culture of United Kingdom science needs a sea-change, in favour of open and positive communication with the media. This will require training and resources; above all it will require leadership ... It will inevitably

involve occasional embarrassment or frustration. But, if it succeeds, it will pay for itself many times over in renewed public trust.

It was to deliver on these recommendations that the idea of the Science Media Centre was born.

***

While MMR and GM were playing out in the headlines, I was working as Head of Press for the Catholic Agency for Overseas Development (CAFOD). I had great fun in the run-up to the millennium with a leading role in the aid agency's Jubilee 2000 campaign for debt relief. In the short term the campaign galvanised an existing desire within both the public and the media to make a grand and meaningful gesture that would make the world a better place. But as the hangovers faded after the millennium celebrations, so too did media interest in developing-world debt. It was getting harder and harder to generate interest in straightforward development issues.

My media strategies became increasingly desperate: I took flood victims from Yorkshire to meet flood victims in Mozambique; dumped gold bullion outside Downing Street to protest at the International Monetary Fund's refusal to sell off gold reserves to fund debt relief; and arranged for the recently converted Catholic MP Ann Widdecombe to visit CAFOD's projects in Africa in the hope of changing her mind about debt relief. The visit did not go well for me. Widdecombe's view that debt relief would enrich corrupt African leaders only hardened during her visit and, on her return, she did a round of radio and TV interviews to say so. When the *Daily Telegraph* op-ed editor told me he would happily take a piece from my director but only if I replaced his name with that of a celebrity like Bob Geldof or Bono, I knew it was time to move on. I needed to work in a field that didn't require a quirky photo call or a celebrity to get some media attention, and when I looked at what had been making headlines, I realised that field was science.

My friends scoffed when I told them I wanted to do media relations for science. My A Levels were in Welsh, English and History, and I had a degree in journalism. But like others at that time, I was fascinated by the debates around GM and MMR, and I was very pro-science. I also wanted to be able to make a difference on issues that were in the headlines but often reported badly.

It was around this time that I read a January 2001 interview with Professor Susan Greenfield in the *Financial Times* in which she discussed her plans to set up a new independent media centre at the Royal Institution to bridge the gap between scientists and journalists. Greenfield was a flamboyant neuroscientist and populariser of science who had recently become the Institution's first female director. Known for her willingness to pose for *Hello!* magazine in her trademark miniskirts as well as her ability to enthral huge crowds with her explanation of how the brain works, she was determined to shake things up. When Lord Sainsbury asked if the Royal Institution would play host to the new media centre recommended in his Lords report, she jumped at the chance.

Six months later, I found myself sitting in front of an intimidating interview panel of eight eminent figures in science including: Greenfield herself, who had by this point been made a baroness by Tony Blair; Dr Philip Campbell, editor-in-chief of *Nature*; and Professor Sir John Krebs, former head of the Natural Environment Research Council. I was the wild-card candidate but that meant I had the advantage of having nothing to lose. I knew I didn't have the scientific qualifications they wanted, but back in 2001, I doubted anyone had the combination of media and hard science they were after. My approach was to argue that what they really needed was someone who combined a deep understanding of the needs of the media with the ability to help scientists speak English. The last thing they needed was an academic. The gamble paid off. Just to drive home the point that they were taking a risk, they offered me the job on £10,000 less than the advertised annual salary, suggesting that they would divert that money into recruiting someone with a PhD. I didn't care. I spent the next few days announcing my new job to my incredulous friends. My adventure in the world of science had begun.

***

There has been a revolution in the culture of science in the past two decades, which has seen scientists transformed from remote figures hidden away in their ivory towers to accessible experts central to our national life. The SMC is widely acknowledged as being both a product of and a catalyst for that change. Through the stories in this book, I chart the progress of this quiet revolution, reveal what was happening behind the scenes of some of the most controversial science stories of the past twenty years, and share my concerns about the new threats facing science communication. We are now familiar with what really happens behind closed doors in politics, thanks to inside stories from spin doctors and special advisers such as Alastair Campbell and Dominic Cummings. The same cannot be said of science, but it clearly has a profound impact on our lives, particularly as we continue to grapple with a world profoundly changed by Covid-19. As a science press officer who has watched from ringside as the worlds of science and the media have collided, I hope that this book will make compelling reading for anyone interested in some of the big science questions of our day or in the complex intersection of science with politics, culture, and society at large.

Some of the stories may be familiar to people of a certain age. Some of you, for example, will recall reading about the October 2009 sacking of Professor David Nutt as the government's chief drugs adviser (Chapter 5), or just a month later, the global furore when climate sceptics seized on an academic's hacked emails as proof that climate science was a hoax (Chapter 6). Other chapters tell bigger stories such as the remarkable transformation of animal testing from science's dirty little secret to a broadly accepted element of medical research (Chapter 2), or how the GM researchers who ran away from sensationalised headlines on 'Frankenstein foods' became the cheerleaders for a new form of media engagement, even when that meant doing battle with Prince Charles and environmental campaigners (Chapter 1). Then there is the story of how the government's attempt to ban research on human–animal embryos led to an unprecedented fightback from scientists and patient advocates (Chapter 4). This laid the basis for future battles for the hearts and minds of politicians and the public on ethically complex issues such as human genome editing and so-called 'three-parent babies'.

Two of the chapters move away from specific science stories and focus on the topics of science communication and journalism more broadly. In Chapter 9, I describe how, despite the SMC's remit and our many battles with the media, I have become a huge champion of the UK's science, health and environment journalists and am often at odds with scientists making lazy generalisations about poor reporting. And in Chapter 10, I talk about my fears that science press officers have become an endangered species, as research-intensive universities become ever more like businesses and research comms get swallowed up within their huge marketing departments.

Not all the stories I have been involved in have ended positively or fit neatly into a wider theme – or arguably even our specific remit – but they cannot be left out. The SMC did relatively little on the controversy that arose when Nobel Prize-winning biologist Sir Tim Hunt made sexist remarks at a science journalism conference in 2015, but I ended up advising him in what became a major global science story (Chapter 8). Conversely, the bitter row over research into myalgic encephalomyelitis (ME), also known as chronic fatigue syndrome, is not an issue most readers will have heard about, but it contains important lessons about what we do at the SMC when research evidence and scientists come under sustained attack (Chapter 3).

The underlying theme of much of the book is that the gains of the revolution in openness need to be vigorously defended. In particular you will find stories about my repeated hard-fought battles against government moves to restrict independent scientists from speaking publicly – from the proposed anti-lobbying clause to the excessive control exerted by government comms officers over independent science communication.

***

Unlike Alastair Campbell, I never anticipated writing a book, and have not kept diaries. As a result, these stories are my own recollections of events that have happened over a period of twenty years. I have no doubt that my version of events will differ in important ways from the recollections of others who lived through them; and am equally sure that – despite my best efforts – my memories will not always be accurate. I apologise now to anyone who feels overlooked or misrepresented in these chapters. When I recently told a Home Office press officer that I was writing about the sacking of Professor David Nutt, he suggested I check that my version of events accorded with his. I politely declined his offer. This book is not intended to be an objective record of science in the media during the twenty-first century: it is my account of my time in it. Or to put it another way – this is my book, and all the things in it are what I remember. Mostly, it is about the people and the stories that touched, angered or inspired me, and the lessons learned from each, now embodied both by our centre and the network of SMCs around the world.

As someone who encourages scientists to emphasise the caveats and limitations of their work, let me add a few more. The media is a broad term used to cover very different kinds of journalism, including news and current affairs, features, documentaries, investigations and so on. As implied by our strapline – 'where science meets the headlines' – the SMC is focused primarily on news and current affairs, and this book reflects that. I am a great fan of investigative journalism and wish there was more of it in science, but the SMC is a small team of eight and our hands are full dealing with a 24/7 news beast that needs constant feeding.

Secondly the SMC does not claim the credit for the changes in the culture of science communication we have seen in the past two decades. In 2002 many doors had already been opened to us by organisations such as the Committee for the Public Understanding of Science and following incentives by funding bodies to reward scientists doing media work. This cultural revolution had well and truly begun; we came along as enthusiastic volunteers to man the barricades.

And a quick note on terminology: this book is a homage to specialist journalists – 'beat' reporters as they used to be called, who focus on one subject, gaining in-depth understanding and insight over many years. In my world these are the science, health, medical and environmental reporters, and they cover different kinds of stories. For ease of reading, I have included them all under the umbrella term of science journalists.

Similarly the SMC works with a wide range of experts, including social scientists and engineers. The latter have often lobbied us to change our name to the Science and Engineering Media Centre. We have resisted because there are no 'engineering journalists' and the media treats engineers as we do – as a critically important group of experts for certain stories. I have generally included them throughout as part of the broad category of SMC experts. On the whole, engineering tends to be seen as less controversial than science,which may be why engineers are sometimes neglected by the media. They are rarely accused of playing God or exposing society to new risks. My response to frustrated engineers who ask us for help in raising their media profile is, be careful what you wish for.

***

I did not set out to become a campaigner for openness in science or to spend so much of my time arguing for a separation of science from government communication. But the SMC's philosophy and outlook have emerged from the stories we got involved with and the battles we fought. If we are more strident than some about the need for scientists to be free from institutional constraints, it's because we have seen how these restrictions can take experts out of the public debate when they are most needed. People often ask me for evidence that such restrictions are harmful to the public. That is hard to prove, and for every scientist prevented from speaking to the media others are thankfully able and willing to help. But I hope that by the end of the book readers will agree with me that allowing more of the UK's scientists to speak to the media can only be good for our national discourse.

When I joined the SMC, I assumed I would spend some years in science before moving on. But twenty years later, I am still here. When I set out, the narrative of science in the media was one of a culture clash between two fields that were once described as 'poor bedfellows'. Quentin Cooper, presenter of BBC Radio 4's

Material World, once attempted to explain why tensions between the two were inevitable: 'Science values detail, precision, the impersonal, the technical, the lasting, facts, numbers and being right. Journalism values brevity, approximation, the personal, the colloquial, the immediate, stories, words and being right now.'

But in an organisation set up precisely because of this clash of cultures, I found something in science that mirrors what I most value about journalism. The scientific method and the journalistic principle of impartiality are both mechanisms aimed at rising above bias and politics to reveal facts and truths that can be conveyed to the public. Such an idealised version of science and the media will be seen as horribly naive by readers who see both disciplines failing to live up to these standards on a daily basis. Others actively want science to embrace politics and disagree with me that this can undermine public trust. But I am sticking to my view that the aspiration, embodied in both science and journalism, of seeking objective and impartial information is needed more than ever in our polarised post-truth world.

People who dislike what the SMC does love to point out that I joined a far-left revolutionary group in my college days, and imply that I have brought some kind of political agenda into the world of science. The first bit of this is true. I did become a communist at college and was politically active for several years. The second bit, however, is not. Unlike some of my former comrades, I was never a very dedicated communist and always much more interested in pursuing a career in media relations.

Far from bringing any political views into science, I have become ever more convinced that science should try hard to maintain a clear separation from politics. Many will say that this is also naive, but I feel that one of the USPs of science is that the scientific method and its associated rigour mean that the public can trust the integrity of research.

In 2013, I was contacted by the honours committee to ask if I would accept an OBE for my services to science. Most people would not have to think twice before proudly accepting. For me, things were not so straightforward. I had met my husband-to-be, a proud Belfast republican, on a protest outside the BBC against the broadcast ban on Gerry Adams. When the offer arrived, we had a short conversation in which he confirmed that he would not leave me if I accepted, but asked that I never mention it in front of him again. It was a deal. As the saying goes, OBE should really stand for 'Other Buggers' Efforts', and I appreciated the recognition it brought for the work of the whole SMC team, past and present, and for science press officers everywhere who rarely get recognised. I also knew that it was nothing to do with approval by the British Empire, and everything to do with the science honours committee.

***

This book was largely written in a short sabbatical in the summer of 2019. The original plan was to get it out by the summer of 2020. But my book about science in the media was put on hold because of the biggest science story of our times – the Covid pandemic. Returning to my draft after an exhausting and often overwhelming eighteen months, I was struck by how the huge cultural changes I relay in this book had prepared the scientific community for a story like no other. Scientific controversies such as Climategate, GM foods or the 'statin wars' had all been a training ground for Covid. The public need for scientists to engage with them via the news media had never been greater. Lives depended on it, as people looked to science for answers about vaccines, mask-wearing, social contact with others, the safety of schools and much more. The idea that science communication was a niche or trivial part of working in science, far less important than the actual proper business of being a scientist, gave way to my vision – that communicating science to the public is a vital, central part of being a great scientist.

1

THE GM WARS

How scientists fought the 'Frankenfoods' narrative

I ONCE WATCHED Tim Radford, the *Guardian*'s former science editor, tell a room full of eminent plant scientists that they should have enjoyed the media feeding frenzy on the dangers of GM crops during the late 1990s. He argued that headlines like 'Frankenstein Foods Horror' had offered researchers a God-given opportunity to explain the science behind this new plant-breeding technique to an engaged but worried public. Looking out at the audience I could see the bewildered scientists trying to process this alien message. Seeing their work presented as a scare story had been their worst nightmare. Of course, Radford was right – they may not have wanted to see GM on the front page of every red top, but once it was there, the best thing to do was to embrace it. Unfortunately, few saw it that way at the time – and their reluctance to engage with the media had disastrous consequences for their work.

GM foods are produced from organisms that have had changes introduced into their DNA through genetic engineering as opposed to traditional cross-breeding. The first GM food approved for release in the USA in 1994 was called Flavr Savr – a tomato variety produced by US company Calgene, and sold as a paste in UK supermarkets. The tomato was genetically engineered to have a longer shelf life and by all accounts proved popular with consumers. The arrival of this new technology in the 1990s had been met with a furious reaction from campaigning bodies such as Greenpeace and Friends of the Earth, which saw GM as a risk to human health and the environment as well as an opportunity for huge multinationals like agricultural giant Monsanto to consolidate their control of the food chain.

Newspaper headlines like 'GM Food "threatens the planet" and 'Is GM the New Thalidomide?' became par for the course. When then prime minister Tony Blair came out in support of GM, he was variously portrayed by the press as the Grim Reaper or Frankenstein. Public concern mounted as the headlines piled up. In March 1998, the supermarket chain Iceland announced that it would ban all GM foods; other UK chains soon followed. In 1999, Prince Charles made his opposition to GM known. The *Daily Mail* led with 'Charles: My fears over the safety of GM foods'. The prince spoke for those who didn't like the idea of meddling with 'natural' food and objected that scientists were taking 'mankind into realms that belong to God and to God alone'. In Alastair Campbell's diaries of the period, the spin doctor reveals that he advised the PM to stop advocating for the technology.

Campbell's diaries also reveal that he suggested to Blair that it ought to be the scientists making the case for GM, not the politicians. The problem was that the UK's mild-mannered plant scientists were ill-equipped for the job. These were the days when most scientists were media shy. Plant scientists had always been the poor relation to medical researchers in terms of media interest, so the sudden and unprecedented demand to go head-to-head with media-savvy non-governmental organisations was completely bewildering to most GM researchers. Some rose to the task, but most ran in the opposite direction, only to then watch in despair as their area of science was repeatedly misrepresented in the news.

Meanwhile, scientific evidence to support the judicious use of GM was mounting. The Farm Scale Evaluations on GM in 2003, the report from the Advisory Committee on Releases to the Environment in 2004, and a major report by the chief scientific adviser to the UK government in 2004 all built on the global scientific consensus that GM was safe and, when used carefully, need not have a negative impact on the environment. Our challenge at the SMC was to persuade plant scientists that it wasn't enough to do the research; they also needed to get out there and talk about it.

Our first significant encounter with the GM story was inauspicious. It ended with the editor of a national newspaper calling for my head on a plate and me believing that my adventure in science had come to an inglorious end just months after it had started.

It began in 2002 with a call from Dr Mark Tester, a senior lecturer in plant biology from the University of Cambridge who had been working on drought-resistant GM crops. Tester explained that he had been involved as an adviser on a forthcoming TV drama called *Fields of Gold* for the BBC, co-written by then-editor of the *Guardian* Alan Rusbridger and scriptwriter Ronan Bennett. The plot followed the fictional story of a young photographer, played by Anna Friel, who discovers that a GM superbug is killing elderly people and wildlife and threatening global havoc. Like most of the plant scientists I had met, Tester was a *Guardian*-reading environmentalist and had been pleased to be recommended as a scientific adviser by Tim Radford.

But this initial pleasure had evaporated when Tester returned from an extended trip to his home country of Australia to find the final rushes of the two-part drama on his doorstep. The viewing was not a happy one. Tester felt the film-makers had either ignored his advice or stretched what he said was theoretically plausible to support a sensationalised storyline. He feared the drama would encourage uninformed anti-GM hysteria. Having contacted the production team to request some changes, Tester was told that he had missed the deadline and he was now horrified that his name was going to be associated with the drama. At first, I urged him to relax. It was only a drama after all, and discerning viewers should be trusted to see it as such. But Tester was determined to put on record that the science was sensational and inaccurate. I suggested an opinion piece in a broadsheet and that perhaps the *Guardian* – despite its links to the drama – would be the best home for it. I reasoned that although the paper probably would not welcome the fact that the main scientific adviser wanted to distance himself from it, it might feel it was smart to give him the space to do so. I therefore sent an email to Tim Radford, suggesting that given that Tester was keen to write something, it might be better published there than in rival papers who would be only too pleased to 'have a pop at the *Guardian*'. It proved to be a fateful email.

In the meantime, alarm bells were ringing elsewhere. My initial argument that we should take a relaxed attitude to a TV drama was not chiming with the scientists and press officers who had been working hard for several years – with little success – to get a more accurate representation of GM crops in the UK press. Bob Ward, who led the media team at the Royal Society, and Ray Mathias, Head of Science Communication at the John Innes Centre, a world-class plant science research institute based in Norwich, had been contacted by the BBC and told that the broadcaster wanted the film to prompt a wider discussion on GM. Producers wanted scientists to take part in a web debate immediately after each episode aired. A great idea, but it showed that the BBC was not treating this as just a standard Saturday night drama – there were no expert debates after *Spooks*! One BBC employee told Mark Tester that the drama would 'show the GM conspiracy as it really is', while the corporation's website declared that one of the aims of the drama was 'tapping into a very real fear, to make people think about what they eat'. As the broadcast date approached, Rusbridger was quoted as saying that *Fields of Gold* 'will – if it succeeds – engage a mass audience and make them question the issues behind it'. Even the actors were buying into the educational aspects of the drama. Max Beesley, who played the heroic anti-GM farmer, told the *Daily Express*: 'People are going to think it's sensationalism because it's television, but I think that it's very close to what actually goes on.'

With concern growing among scientists, I felt under pressure to do something. I still didn't want to overreact, but equally waiting passively to see what impact it might have was probably not the bold and proactive approach the scientific community was hoping for from the SMC. Then I had an idea. Thanks to Dr Tester, we had a copy of the drama. Why not invite scientists to watch a private screening of the film, get their responses and circulate them in advance? It seemed in line with our mission to move scientists onto the front foot.

We bought the popcorn and invited ten eminent plant scientists and their press officers to a film show. Our sole interest was in the science that drove the plot – specifically the central idea that the effects of GM could jump across species from crops to animals to humans – so I urged the scientists to limit their comments to what was scientifically plausible rather than comment on the quality of the acting or cinematography. After several years of bruising headlines, they did not hold back. Professor Phil Mullineaux from the John Innes Centre described it as 'the BBC's answer to the *X-Files*, where the science is complete fantasy'. Many of them lamented a missed opportunity for a nuanced debate about this complex issue.

By far the strongest statement came from Lord May, president of the Royal Society, the UK's national academy of science, and former chief scientific adviser to the UK government. He hadn't been able to join us at the SMC showing, but watched it later that day. He did not mince his words:

> This ludicrous piece of alarmist science fiction, which is presented as a realistic examination of the issues surrounding GM, is a disgrace . . . This hysterically inaccurate treatment of an important and many-sided public issue shows the same lack of sensitivity as, say, a drama that portrayed asylum-seekers as murderous aliens from Mars. The BBC will be abdicating its responsibility to its viewers by broadcasting this error-strewn piece of propaganda, which most certainly does not help to promote informed public debate around the issues.

With the *Guardian* seemingly not keen to run Mark Tester's piece, after some discussion with the other press officers involved, we agreed to send the responses to science correspondents at the *Daily Telegraph* and *The Times* – papers perceived by scientists we were working with at the time as having a track record of accurate reporting on GM. The next day was a shock to me, so I can only imagine how it felt to Alan Rusbridger. The two papers had splashed the 'row' on their front pages. I knew I had inadvertently waded into something bigger than the science of GM when Roger Highfield, then science editor of the *Telegraph*, called up later that day saying his editors wanted more. I was later told that for Charles Moore, the conservative and 'unionist' editor of the *Telegraph*, the criticism of *Fields of Gold* was a double delight as Ronan Bennett, Rusbridger's co-author on the drama, was a former Irish Republican who had once been accused of and briefly imprisoned for shooting a policeman in Belfast. I told him there was nothing more to offer and that neither we nor the scientists were interested in using this against the *Guardian*. I spent much of that day avoiding the phone. If it wasn't *The Times* and the *Telegraph* wanting more, it was the rest of the press yelling at me for not giving them the story. The scientists meanwhile were thrilled. Lord May, who had been sceptical about the establishment of the SMC, sent me a congratulatory note to say that he could now see what our purpose was.

Any sense of achievement on my part, however, was short-lived. Soon after I turned on *Newsnight* to see Rusbridger claiming that the SMC was a sinister, pro-biotech 'lobby group' with an axe to grind against the *Guardian*. He referenced the email I had sent to Tim Radford, claiming it proved that the SMC had an anti-*Guardian* agenda as I was offering the criticisms around as a terrific story for anyone wanting to dump on the BBC and the *Guardian*. The following week, the *Guardian*'s sister paper the *Observer* ran a piece by Ronan Bennett attacking the scientific community's response to the drama. Under the headline 'The conspiracy to undermine the truth about our GM drama', Bennett described the SMC as the 'lobbying organisation' behind the story and singled out the industry supporters from our list of donors without acknowledging others. 'Its funders include DuPont, Merlin Biosciences, Pfizer, PowderJect and Smith & Nephew – all biotech or pharmaceutical companies with a direct interest in the promotion of the technologies the drama explores.' Bennett claimed that Mark Tester had changed his mind about his scientific advice, a claim Tester denied, and argued that scientific opinion remained deeply divided over GM.

The next day I called Steve Connor, then science editor of the *Independent*, offering him my version of events to ensure it was in the public domain. None of this felt like fun. It was May. The SMC had only opened its doors in April. The words of Alastair Campbell were ringing in my ears – you have really fucked up when the press officer becomes the story.

In June, Rusbridger wrote a three-page letter to my employers at the Royal Institution, Britain's eminent science research body, raising questions about my role and my suitability for the job:

> Ms Fox was, as I am sure you aware, a contributor to *Living Marxism* ... a magazine and movement which grew out of the Revolutionary Communist Party. Her sister, Claire, remains a director and leading figure within the group. This was an organisation which praised the IRA and Saddam Hussein, defended the right of racists publicly to deny that the Holocaust occurred while comparing environmentalists to Nazis ... I would be interested to learn whether she has disclosed these facts to her board.

The Royal Institution passed the letter to the SMC's board to deal with and I spent a nervous few weeks wondering how the board members would react. Rusbridger's theory that my work on *Fields of Gold* was motivated by a malign political agenda sounded plausible. And I don't doubt he believed it. But it wasn't true. Nothing that had happened in those few weeks had anything to with my past involvement in radical left politics. Every decision had been made alongside my immediate colleagues in the SMC and scientists and press officers from leading research institutes. At the next board meeting, I offered to leave the room while they decided my fate. The board did not feel the need. They had examined everything we had done and were satisfied that Rusbridger's complaint was a classic case of shooting the messenger. I lived to fight another day.

I did, however, have my own nagging doubts about whether we had strayed too close to the kind of media campaigns I had been involved with in my previous roles for organisations such as CAFOD. Working for an overseas aid agency desperate to get the media interested in developing-world issues had made me especially accomplished at media campaigning and PR stunts. With hindsight I certainly felt that offering the GM story to only two newspapers had been the wrong decision and had fuelled Rusbridger's suspicion that there was a more sinister agenda at play. My reservations stimulated a good discussion about the positioning of the SMC. Were we to become a sort of Greenpeace for science or adopt a more cautious approach more in line with mainstream science? We decided to tread more carefully in future.

In the event, nothing quite like this has ever happened since, so it's hard to judge how we would handle such a scenario today. Maybe we would ask scientists to watch the programme when it aired and then send their reactions to all news outlets at same time. But it's worth saying that the science press officers we worked with back then felt a sense of deep satisfaction that the viewing public could enjoy an entertaining Saturday night drama safe in the knowledge that the UK's best plant scientists felt it was more akin to science fiction than science fact.

It is also worth pointing out that *Fields of Gold* aired at a time when the *Guardian* was seen by some in science as an anti-GM newspaper. Exactly a year later in April 2003, I was a guest at the launch of *Life*, the paper's new science supplement. Its contributors included Ian Sample, James Randerson, Alok Jha and David Adam – all excellent science reporters who had cut their teeth on specialist titles such as *New Scientist* and *Nature News*. They all remained on the paper after *Life* closed and the *Guardian*'s science coverage remains among the best. Maybe there were positives for both the SMC and the newspaper from the events surrounding the drama, even if it was a bruising experience on all sides.

My next major encounter with GM came hot on the heels of this first one, but thankfully it involved the SMC doing something it was much more comfortable with – supporting scientists to get the best possible media coverage for important scientific findings on a controversial trial. It was Professor Chris Pollock who initiated our involvement by asking me for a meeting in the summer of 2002 to discuss the findings of the Farm Scale Evaluations (FSEs) – a five-year-long series of field trials designed to test whether GM had a negative impact on biodiversity.

The trials had started back in 1998, when three types of genetically modified herbicide-tolerant (GMHT) crops (beet, spring oilseed rape and maize) were on the verge of entering commercial agriculture in the UK. They had passed most of the government's regulatory risk-assessment procedures, which focused on genetic stability and gene-flow issues, but there were concerns about their impact on the environment. English Nature, the government's own advisory body, raised fears about the potential future role that GMHT crops would have, if commercialised, on already-struggling farmland wildlife. Several ecology studies had identified the intensification of agriculture since the 1950s as the major reason for the decline measured in farmland wildlife. Many organisations and environmental scientists were legitimately concerned that the herbicide management of GMHT crops in commercial use would further exacerbate a decline in wildlife if they encouraged very strong levels of weed control, which in turn would reduce invertebrate and bird numbers.

It was in response to these concerns that in October 1998 Michael Meacher MP, then minister of state for the environment, announced the FSE trials. Importantly, the trials were never intended to study gene flow or food safety, both of which had already been assessed and deemed to present a sufficiently low risk to human health and the environment to allow commercialisation. The core purpose of the FSEs was to establish whether the management of GM crops had a perceptibly greater impact on wildlife compared with standard crops.

Professor Pollock, who was a leading figure in GM science and director of the respected Institute of Grassland and Environmental Research in Aberystwyth, had been appointed as chair of the FSE steering group and I had been in touch with him right from the very earliest days of the SMC. In fact, in his typically straight-talking fashion, he had been quick to communicate his reservations about our approach with *Fields of Gold* and was keen for us to focus more on helping plant scientists facilitate better-quality reporting on GM research. Valuing his input, I was all too happy to accept his request for a meeting in the summer of 2002.

Before either of us had even taken a sip of tea Pollock expressed his discontent with the Department for Environment, Food & Rural Affairs (Defra), declaring, 'Defra press office is handling this story over my dead body.' Instead he wanted the SMC to handle the announcement and press briefing for the results of the FSE trials, working with the scientists involved to prepare them for speaking to the media. He had got my attention. The professor went on to say that poor media handling by Defra, political meddling by Meacher, and the anti-GM editorial stance of many of the big newspapers had meant that the public had never really seen balanced and accurate reporting of the experiment. That pained him. His modest request was that the hundreds of ecologists who had worked so hard on the trials would get to have their say when the results were published. I was in.

Professor Pollock was not only a great researcher. He also embodied the philosophy of science that I fell in love with, especially the need for science to resist politicisation and to strive to achieve impartiality. One of the phrases he used when explaining why he did not want political interference or spin in the communication of the FSE trials was: 'If it's not open, it's not science.' It is a phrase that has had a huge influence on our approach.

The results of the trials were due to be published in 2003 in the *Proceedings of the Royal Society* and I found the months of preparation for publication fascinating. I spent a day at one of the trial sites and marvelled at the low-tech nature of their experiments. How do you test whether a GM crop damages biodiversity? Well, you literally collect, identify and count the number of bugs in the GM fields and then compare and contrast them with the equivalent figures from conventional fields. It amused me that even the ecologists didn't always recognise the insects captured in white plastic pots and had to consult a huge bug field guide to check what some of them were.

The tension mounted as the publication date approached. There was a lot riding on these results for both sides in the 'GM wars', with people hoping they would be either a green light or the death knell for the controversial new technology. By that time, the authors knew the scientific results were, as so often, not going to be that clear cut. For two of the three crops (beet and rape), the level of biodiversity was found to be higher in the fields of conventional plants than in the GM ones. But for the third crop (maize), it was the other way round – the level was higher in the fields of GM plants than in the conventional ones. To add to the complexity, the difference in biodiversity was significantly bigger between different types of crop, regardless of whether they were GM or non-GM varieties.

If reported in a fair and measured way, the trials represented neither the green light nor the death knell, which is exactly the kind of complexity and nuance the media hates. My job was to help prepare the scientists to present the findings clearly and accessibly and to anticipate the main questions from the media. I have never been a big fan of tightly controlled press conferences and am wary of the 'key messages' and 'agreed lines' beloved of many PR officers. At the SMC we prefer to encourage authors to stick to the science and go for maximum openness. Critically, preparation for our press conferences involves ensuring that scientists are not hyping their findings and doing everything possible to maximise the chances of measured and accurate coverage. I also tried to prepare them for the backlash from anti-GM campaigners and for the high chance that some journalists would go straight to campaigners and lead with their reaction. If the data had shown a clear result against GM, the scientists would probably have been lauded by anti-GM campaigners. But the more ambiguous findings would prompt lots of criticism of the trial. I was also wary of the reverse: pro-GM campaigners trying to spin the findings as strong evidence in favour of GM. The goal was to generate coverage that reflected the nuanced scientific findings in the context of accurate reporting of the trials themselves.

The results of the study were under embargo – a long-standing 'gentleman's agreement' whereby journalists are allowed to see results a day or two before the time and date that they are officially published. Both science and the media benefit from the embargo system. Ensuring that the world's media all publish a story at exactly the same time means you can dramatically improve its visibility and impact, while also giving reporters time to check facts, set up filming and interviews, speak to authors and approach third-party experts.

On this occasion, however, the *Guardian* splashed the key findings on the front page days before the embargo lifted. When we contacted the paper asking it to take the report down, it claimed that no embargo had been broken and it had been sent a leaked copy of the paper. I disagreed. All the science and environment reporters knew the paper was going to be published in an embargoed journal and launched at an embargoed press conference. It was not the first or last time we would disagree with journalists on what constitutes a broken embargo, but it was the first test of an approach that I had brought with me into science – never reward a newspaper for breaking an embargo by lifting it, thereby sacrificing your entire media strategy and the months of preparation for a press launch. Despite other journalists yelling down the phone at me that we had to lift the embargo, I persuaded the scientists and the journal to hold their nerve. We issued a statement pointing out that the leaked findings were an early draft and therefore not accurate and confirmed that the press briefing would go ahead as planned.

The day before the conference, scientists arrived for a practice event hosted in the SMC. We had decided that wine was in order and by the time the mock briefing was coming to an end several of us were quite merry. The next morning, I poked my head around the doors of the beautiful and historic library at the Royal Institution to see a room full of familiar faces – mostly science and environment reporters, who tended to cover GM more responsibly and accurately than their colleagues in politics and consumer affairs. The press briefing was reserved for these journalists, our standard policy to ensure that scientists could present their findings directly to the press and respond to their questions, without being diverted by other stakeholders wanting to grandstand or ask longer, more convoluted questions. The media could and would go to third parties after the press briefing. Then word reached the green room that Michael Meacher had turned up and walked straight past the press officer on the door.

Although Meacher had commissioned the FSEs, he was regarded with suspicion by scientists. They resented the fact that he was openly anti-GM when they felt he should have been neutral, and they suspected him of leaking secret details about the research to members of Greenpeace and the Soil Association. With minutes to spare, and preferring to deal with the minister before the press conference rather than during it, I dashed off to find him, took a deep breath and asked him to leave. He was extremely displeased but obliged, which was just as well because I didn't have a plan B. I personally escorted him down the Royal Institute's iconic staircase and on to the street. Only then did I realise that I had been filmed by several camera crews. Fortunately, throwing Meacher out of a press conference did my reputation no harm within the scientific community.

The press conference went beautifully. The journalists asked probing questions but listened carefully to the answers. It was exactly what the scientists had wanted – their day in court to explain the science to a group of journalists who were keen to report what they had learned. Predictably some of the next day's headlines were negative, reflecting the narrative of the previous reporting. But underneath the headlines, the articles themselves were much more nuanced than previous coverage and included quotes and facts from the conference.

Despite the success of the media work around the FSEs, however, the wider debate about GM raged on for several more years. One problem with working in news is that it's hard to escape. Building sandcastles with my young son on a beach in France in the summer of 2008, I caught sight of a gentleman reading the *Daily Telegraph*. The front page carried a large photograph of Prince Charles under the heading 'Earth faces GM catastrophe, warns Prince'. In this exclusive interview with journalist Jeff Randall, he pinned the blame for environmental disaster and global warming on GM. I brushed off the sand and called the office. My colleagues were already absorbed in that heady mix of anger and exhilaration that often comes with breaking news on a contentious story.

While some eminent plant scientists and press officers were delighted to give us comments on Charles's outburst, others worried that taking on the future king was unwise. As is often the case at the SMC, our job that morning was to encourage scientists to be bold and to dissuade risk-averse science press officers from reining them in. We had no view on what these scientists should say about the prince's comments, but we were sure that they should say something. In August's 'silly season', when Parliament is closed for the holidays and more serious policy stories are rare, this was huge news, and the public was watching. The result was, frankly, a joy to witness. Several years earlier, many scientists I had met while setting up the SMC had admitted to keeping their heads down and avoiding the press during past scientific controversies. Now they were openly challenging Prince Charles's comments as erroneous and biased. Within twenty-four hours, the headlines had completely changed. 'Prince Charles accused by scientists of abusing his position over GM food,' said the *Daily Telegraph*. 'Scientists condemn Prince Charles's attack on GM crops,' said the *Guardian*. By championing a new way of doing things, we were transforming what the public saw and heard.

Our role was not simply to help the scientists; we also helped journalists to interpret new findings on GM. I recall taking a call from ITV's science and medical editor Lawrence McGinty in September 2012 that appeared to signal a potentially explosive new chapter in the GM story. Back in 1998, a scientist called Dr Árpád Pusztai gave an extended interview on an episode of *World in Action* in which he claimed that rats fed on a diet of GM potatoes suffered stunted growth and problems with their immune systems. The claims were later published in the *Lancet* and repeated throughout the media for the following twelve months at the height of the GM frenzy, with little challenge from scientists. Science, it seemed, had taken a crucial step towards proving the worst predictions from the campaigners – that GM would damage human health. The scientific community responded by announcing a Royal Society special inquiry, which reported in June 1999 – almost an entire year after Pusztai had made his claims. The findings were clear and damning: 'The GM study conducted by Pusztai and the Rowett Institute had major design flaws. There is no convincing evidence supporting adverse health effects from GM potatoes.' If GM does harm humans, this study was most definitely not the one that proved it. The Royal Society's report was bold and robust, but it was also twelve months too late. The long time lag represented what was wrong back then with the scientific community's engagement with ongoing controversies like GM. We needed that same scientific rigour and authority, but in real time.

This was by no means an isolated incident. Much of what goes wrong in the media coverage of science takes place when small or preliminary one-off studies are presented as providing a definitive answer, or when weak results are presented as being significant enough to prompt changes in behaviour or policy. Alzheimer's disease and cancer would have been cured long ago if every small study reported as a 'breakthrough' had in fact been one. Most are not. The SMC identified early on that new findings published in journals are a key area in which science can be misreported. To tackle the issue, we persuaded the press officers of all the biggest science journals to give us early sight of the papers they had decided to press release each week so that we could collect comments from third-party scientists to help journalists put the new findings in context, highlighting any caveats or limitations.

It was surprising, then, when Lawrence McGinty called to say that he had an embargoed study on his hands that we knew nothing about. McGinty explained it was by a French scientist called Professor Gilles-Éric Séralini and showed that rats fed on GM foods developed cancer in a two-year feeding trial. This was explosive – all the more so for coming from a figure like McGinty, who had come to ITN from *New Scientist*, an unusual route for a national TV news journalist. No science stories got on ITN news without his say-so. Was this finally the evidence that GM kills? While the SMC's role is to guide journalists to where the scientific consensus lies on GM, MMR and climate change, we will always be ready to publicise any good-quality study that comes along to overturn that consensus. This was exciting, and whichever way it went, we were needed.

Then things got weird. McGinty explained that the PR agency that sent him the press release had requested he sign a non-disclosure agreement that would prevent him from sharing the full paper with the SMC or any third-party scientists. Cue one of my sweary rants to colleagues. What decent scientist would stop journalists from seeking third-party comments about new findings? I smelt a rat (if you'll pardon the pun). Several hurried calls to other journalists revealed that many had also received the paper and had signed the NDA, and none felt able to send us the paper even though they wanted to find out whether the research was sound. We were desperate. The world's media were about to report a study claiming that GM can cause cancer and we had no way of offering any scientific scrutiny. It felt like a colossal failure.

Just as my swearing levels had gone through the roof, we got news that *L'Observateur*, a French current-affairs magazine, had broken the story before the embargo had been lifted. This allowed the journalists to send us the paper without breaching their NDAs and gave us a few hours to get it out for comments from scientists before a London press conference was scheduled. To help facilitate this process, Professor Maurice Moloney, director of Rothamsted Research, had gathered a group of the institute's scientists to pore over the paper as soon as it arrived. With a London press conference looming and anxious to receive the group's comments, I called the professor about five times in quick succession. Finally, he answered the phone and shouted in his lovely Irish accent: 'If you would stop fecking calling me, we could actually read the paper and send you a comment!' Silence. Then he laughed and so did I. Fair enough.

After an agonising wait, the comments finally started to arrive. We had deliberately reached out beyond plant scientists in our attempts to review the study thoroughly, and comments were also coming in from different universities and research institutes, including toxicologists, statisticians, animal-research experts, food scientists and physiologists. There had been no conferring, but the responses had one thing in common. They all agreed this study was unreliable. Séralini's experiments were too small-scale to draw firm conclusions; he had used the wrong statistical tests; his choice of rat breed skewed the result because the animals were predisposed to tumours, so even the control animals formed them; and he ran the trial much longer than is approved by the suppliers and toxicologists with implications for animal welfare. We sent the responses to the journalists – and waited.

The first response came from Lawrence McGinty himself, who had retreated to the pub across the road from ITN. He was on his first large glass of Chardonnay, having told his editors the story was not worth reporting. Others ran it, but under headlines like 'French GM-fed rat study triggers furore' (BBC), 'Experts criticise GM crop study' (Press Association), and 'Study on Monsanto GM corn concerns draws scepticism' (Reuters). A study may one day emerge that shows GM foods are harmful, but extraordinary claims need extraordinary evidence. This study was not that evidence, and it was critical that the public knew that on the day it was published, not twelve months later.

Later that year, I was invited to speak in the French parliament about the SMC's role in the Séralini story. Unlike the UK, the French media had reported on the study prominently with little or no third-party comment from independent scientists, and public outrage had been such that the French government had been forced to announce a review of its GM policy. Not surprisingly, France's science minister had been intrigued to know why things had played out so differently in the UK. It felt like confirmation of our impact.

These days, I'm pleased to say that the media coverage and tone of the debate around GM in the UK has changed dramatically. There may still be little appetite for GM among the UK public, but the levels of hostility of the late 1990s have all but disappeared and the UK media's coverage is generally more responsible. When we started out, it was often reported by consumer affairs or political journalists more interested in the controversy than the science. Now many of the media stories are written by science journalists reporting on specific new applications of GM, many of which are examples of 'public good' research such as the attempt to make fish oils from plants or the development of vitamin-enriched rice for the developing world. More broadly, many plant scientists are interested in GM as a way of reducing the environmental impacts of intensive and extensive agriculture. Take Professor Giles Oldroyd, for example. As part of his role as director of the Crop Science Centre at the University of Cambridge he conducts research on using GM to grow crops that can produce their own nitrogen fertilisers – a holy grail of plant science. When talking about his work, he deliberately talks about 'organic GM' to make the point to anti-GM campaigners that he and they share similar goals of enhancing sustainability in agriculture and should embrace GM as a way of achieving their aims.

Twenty years on, what did we learn from the 'GM wars'? That both science and society pay a high price when experts retreat from a controversy; that the media narrative can change when scientists take a more proactive approach; and that sometimes you have to play the long game.

2

DON'T MENTION THE A WORD

The long road to openness on animal research

IN 2002, I ARRIVED at the Wellcome Trust's gleaming glass offices on Euston Road for my first meeting on animal research. At the reception desk, as I began to explain what I was there for, a horrified receptionist placed her finger over her lips. Lowering her voice to a whisper, she said: 'We don't mention the A word.'

It was a sentiment I encountered again and again. A cursory glance at the headlines on animal research from that year reveals that media coverage was dominated by the eye-catching and at times illegal activities of animal rights protesters, intent on ending all animal testing, willing to use violence and intimidation to do so, and often sympathetically reported on by non-science journalists. While there had been protests for decades against the use of animals in research, the violence took a turn for the worse in the late 1980s with various home-made bombs used to target institutions and individuals. That set in train the cat-and-mouse decade of the 1990s during which violent protests continued, despite greater coordination across police and security forces.

Today, things look very different. Animal research is no longer science's dirty little secret; it is conducted with much more openness. This has robbed animal rights activists of one of their central accusations: that scientists concealed their animal research because it involved the mistreatment of animals.

The question of animal research is always going to be a particularly controversial one in a nation of animal lovers. And it's undeniable that in the past animal rights groups did expose some genuine (as well as many fictitious) instances of poor animal welfare. Publicising those helped to bring about improvements. The challenge is how to facilitate a well-informed discussion on an endeavour that many people would prefer did not have to happen but that remains a vital necessity for public health. Covid vaccines and drug treatments are only the latest example of this. Yet at the turn of the new millennium there was little possibility of having an informed debate on this issue when the science community refused to talk about this aspect of their work. The solution was, ultimately, to let the light in.

I support openness in science as an important principle in its own right. Sometimes that means helping scientists robustly defend this key aspect of biological science against criticism and explain the rationale to the public. However, openness is not only about defending animal research. Debating the issues candidly in the media is also a means of testing the validity of arguments for animal research, allowing journalists to scrutinise the process, and enabling scientists working with animals to report any bad practice or speak freely about potential reform. When Professor Sir Patrick Bateson was commissioned by the government to do a report on primate research, I wasted no time in lobbying him to launch it at the SMC. When the time came, the report showed that 91 per cent of research on non-human primates between 1997 and 2007 was of high quality and scientifically justified. Quite rightly the media framed the story differently, leading with the shocking number of experiments on monkeys that failed this test. 'One-in-ten monkey experiments unjustified', said Channel 4 News, while the BBC ran with 'Bateson Report: Monkey Research can be improved'. I was pleased to see the report covered in this way – alongside the comprehensive recommendations that Bateson made to avoid that failure rate in future, including a vetting system for primate experiments run by the independent National Centre for the Replacement, Refinement and Reduction of Animals in Research.

There is also a very good argument that transparency is the key to reasoned and sensible media coverage. Hiding whatever is contested and controversial serves only to fuel controversy and suspicion, even when hiding is an understandable response in the face of illegal protest and violence. It was not – and is not – the SMC's job to campaign in support of animal research, and I never saw it that way; our mission is to ensure that the public has easy access to accurate and evidence-based information.

My husband has taught politics and sociology to sixth formers for over twenty years. In his first classes with new students, he encourages them to develop their critical-thinking skills by debating controversial subjects. When the topic of animal research comes up he is often struck by how many students are initially opposed to it, but then change their view when exposed to the arguments. Public opinion polls have also borne this out: most people are instinctively uncomfortable about the prospect of subjecting animals to any pain and discomfort until they understand the role of animal research in the development and testing of medicines that alleviate pain and suffering in both humans and animals, as well as in studying how our modern world affects wild animal populations.

Animal research is an issue that we will need to discuss and debate for as long as it is with us. And it is not black and white.

Biological scientists may broadly support the need to use animals in research but there is plenty of healthy debate within the field about the best ways to do so and much effort is invested in replacing, reducing and refining their use (known as the 3Rs).

Nonetheless, it is undeniable that testing on animals has been involved in the development of almost every medical treatment available today – antibiotics, insulin, cancer drugs, heart surgery and organ transplant. I remember one SMC press briefing in the late 2000s, where scientists reported a small increase in the amount of research conducted on primates in a one-year period. But they were able to tell the assembled journalists that the increase was linked to the approval process for the new 'biological drug' Herceptin. Many newspapers had spent the previous year campaigning for the drug to be licensed – hailing it as a wonder drug for cancer treatment. It was as clear an example as I've seen of the balance between risks and benefits – with the practice of primate research having to be weighed against the delivery of new hope to millions of cancer patients.

There are plenty of valid criticisms to be made about different aspects of animal research, but the aggressive tactics of animal rights extremists have hindered rather than encouraged the open and critical debate that we should have on this issue. When I arrived at the SMC in 2001, I had not quite grasped the extent to which scientists had been encouraged to retreat. I was appalled to find out that most universities and research institutes were quiet about their use of animals as a matter of official policy. Their press releases about studies using animal models generally omitted to mention the fact, university websites made no mention of animal research, individual institutions did not publish the numbers of animals they used, and if a university had an animal lab, you could bet it was housed in a nondescript building with no name. For the SMC – a new centre charged with getting scientists to engage more effectively with topical controversies – this collective silence felt like a major test.

The widespread policy of secrecy was all the more galling when I got to know the handful of scientists who had chosen to buck this trend and speak out about their use of animals in research. Professor Colin Blakemore was the best known. A leading neuroscientist at the University of Oxford, he and his family had been targeted by animal rights protesters because he made use of cats in his work on vision disorders. The campaign against Blakemore was violent and horrible and spanned many years. His daughter Sarah-Jayne Blakemore, now a professor and leading scientist herself, spoke movingly about the impact on their family life in her award-winning book on teenagers:

> The animal rights activists threatened to kidnap me and my two younger sisters, resulting in the three of us, aged between six and eleven at the time, being followed to and from school by undercover police in an unmarked car . . . each time we wanted to drive anywhere, my parents would check under the car with a bomb-detector mirror. Getting in a car that might explode as soon as the ignition was turned on was not an experience I enjoyed much.

Professor Blakemore deeply resented the attempt to terrorise his family, yet he made a conscious decision to continue engaging with the media and the public on animal research. Supported by the Research Defence Society (a lobby group set up by scientists in 1908 to defend the use of animal research to the public and challenge misinformation), he made regular appearances on TV and radio to debate the issues with opponents. He was not the only one to do so, but he was part of a tiny group – the few others included Professor Clive Page from King's College London, Professor

Nancy Rothwell from the University of Manchester, Professor
Tipu Aziz from Oxford, Professor Roger Lemon from University
College London and Professor Max Headley from the University
of Bristol. These scientists got little support from their universities.
At best, they were encouraged to keep their heads down; at worst,
they were abandoned to fight this public battle alone.

The blame for this situation lay with animal rights extremists
who were prepared to use violence and intimidation as a means
to an end. But the collective failure of the scientific community to
stand up for this legitimate area of scientific endeavour was distressing. More importantly, the silence meant that the public were
hearing only one narrative on animal research. Anyone who has
picked up a leaflet from an animal rights activist in a town centre
will know that the images used are almost exclusively of cats, dogs
and monkeys – but what they probably won't know is that there
have been special protections in place for these animals since 1876
preventing their use in most circumstances with the result that
for years they have been involved in fewer than 1 per cent of all
experimental procedures. The photos are also frequently decades
old and/or from overseas, and depict procedures and conditions
that would for decades now not have gained ethical and regulatory
approval in the UK.

The fight for greater transparency on animal research felt as
if it lay at the heart of the SMC's mission. But my views soon pitted me against many of the institutional communications teams
I was trying to court. Press officers who went to great lengths
to get scientists into the news on other subjects would explain
that encouraging them to speak on animal research would put
the institution at risk of attack. Those scientists and press officers
who wanted more openness were outvoted by senior staff who
prioritised caution. But over time, what became glaringly obvious
to me was that a policy of not speaking about animal research

was self-defeating. The scientific community was doing the job of animal rights activists for them. By remaining quiet about the use of animals, scientists and their institutions were making it easier for protesters to present this research as secretive and, by extension, shameful.

I wasn't convinced that the scientists or institutions targeted by animal rights extremists had been identified because they had been open about their use of animals. It seemed to me that the likes of Cambridge, Oxford and Huntingdon Life Sciences had become targets despite decades of keeping their heads down, rather than the opposite. The activists could have chosen their targets through different means. This hunch was confirmed to me by special police units set up to monitor animal rights extremism who found scientific papers in the homes of extremists with the sections on the use of animals highlighted. It wasn't hard for them to find out which scientists were using animals in their research.

'It's ok for you, Fiona, you won't be the one with the bomb under your car,' became a familiar mantra, especially from those cautious senior communications managers at universities and research institutes. It felt like an unbridgeable gap, and I understood why. This kind of violent attack was very rare but the threats were nonetheless frightening, and I empathised with that. Of course no vice-chancellor or head of communications wanted their university to become the next target for extremists. But I firmly believed this was a classic case of strength in numbers. If everyone in UK science whose research relied on animal testing was open about it, they would vastly outnumber the tiny group of animal rights extremists, who lacked the capacity to target more than one or two institutions at a time. And if everyone was open and acknowledged it as a widespread practice, there would then be less justification for the activists to target any one particular scientist.

Being at odds with so many in the scientific community was not comfortable, and I tried hard in those early years at the SMC to understand the reasons for keeping animal research under the radar. But it was my job to consider the impact of this collective silence on public attitudes. Helping turn this situation around was a real test of whether we could make a difference to media relations on topical controversies in science.

The problem was that I wasn't convincing the scientific community. I remember getting my first audience with a pro-vice-chancellor for research at a top London university in 2005. As I entered a huge office with its oak panelling, plush red leather couches and paintings of famous alumni on the walls, I had my killer points rehearsed and was feeling quietly confident. I would point out that the extremists were too few in number to target every university; that universities could provide strength in numbers if more moved towards openness; and that there was no evidence to suggest that either individual scientists or institutions were targeted because they had spoken to the media. To cap it off, I could show that two of his scientists were already speaking out with no ill effect to the university, so supporting them (rather than discouraging them as his media team was then doing) was the right thing to do and not high risk. If I could persuade this guy, we could have a real breakthrough for openness that might start a chain reaction.

To his credit, he gave me almost an hour of his time and listened intently. But at the end, he explained that he could not in all conscience do anything that would make his university the next target for animal rights extremists. The experiences of Cambridge and Oxford were too raw. It would be too disruptive, too expensive. He was sorry, but there would be no change. It was one of many similar meetings that became one of the least enjoyable parts of my early years at the SMC.

Another argument used frequently was that not speaking out on animals was proof of 'showing a duty of care to our scientists'. Like the 'bomb under the car' argument, this had the effect of making it look like those of us arguing for more openness were irresponsible, advocating a policy that jeopardised the safety of researchers. I saw it differently. Hiding animal research implied that the institution was not proud of the research it conducted or prepared to defend it publicly.

In 2012, Imperial College London was infiltrated by an animal rights activist affiliated with the British Union for the Abolition of Vivisection (BUAV – now Cruelty Free International) who worked undercover in one of their animal labs for months, before going to the *Sunday Times* with video footage they claimed revealed serious animal cruelty. I knew from previous BUAV infiltrations that scientists working in these labs had accused the campaign group of editing video footage collected over many months to make routine regulated procedures look sinister and to frame minor lapses in care – similar to anything you might see daily in a hospital ward – to look like animal cruelty.

I lobbied the university press team to invite the newspaper into the lab as we had done successfully when the same thing happened at an animal-breeding company. On that occasion the newspaper had sent their own journalist and photographer who had full access to the facility and the article was much more measured as a result. I was told this was impossible because of the university's duty of care to the researchers – instead, it issued a short corporate statement that avoided answering the specific accusations, and announced an independent inquiry. The *Sunday Times* ran the story in April 2013 along with the video footage and sensational claims that rats had been 'beheaded and had their necks broken'.

I knew the university had the best interests of its scientists at heart and this was a horrible situation. It was possible that the researchers themselves might not have wanted the university to speak out in their defence. But I still questioned whether letting people read unchallenged attacks on these scientists was the best way to deal with this.

Imperial's independent inquiry and a Home Office investigation later published reports. None of the animal cruelty allegations reported by the media were upheld, though the reports did find some lapses in animal welfare procedures and made recommendations to improve the university's ethical review process, management and training. The findings were a far cry from the BUAV claims of 'appalling animal suffering on a very large scale' or 'wholly inadequate care of animals by Imperial staff'. I wrote to other universities and research institutes calling on them to plan for future such undercover infiltrations, and urging them in such circumstances to invite news outlets into their facilities to address key allegations openly. In the event, most mainstream news outlets started to become wary of animal rights groups touting round these videos, and stopped carrying them.

I tried hard not to be glib in dismissing the link between speaking out and becoming a target. I decided to gather data to see whether there was a link between more openness and the targeting of scientists. I was fastidious about following up with scientists who we did persuade to speak to journalists. Time and time again they told us that they had had no problems.

Dr Sarah Bailey, a pharmacologist from the University of Bath, had approached us in summer 2006 to say she was scared to publicise a new study showing for the first time that a controversial anti-acne drug called Roaccutane appeared to cause depressive symptoms in mice. This was one of the first lab studies on an association that was being widely reported – anecdotally – in humans and it was important the findings were reported to the public carefully through the news media. Along with the Bath press office, we persuaded Dr Bailey not to let fear stop her from getting these important findings into the public domain. We ran a mock press briefing with her to prep her for questions on using mice as part of her research. On the day of the press briefing, she described how you can tell that a mouse is depressed, a description she went on to give in numerous broadcast interviews throughout the day.

When I checked in with her in the following days and weeks, she reported that she had received hundreds of emails. Not from animal rights activists, but from the parents of teenagers who had become depressed after taking the drugs. They wanted to thank her for her work. Bailey became a champion for openness on animal research, and still speaks at SMC events to encourage her peers to speak out. I used her experience to remind nervous communications managers that we were not asking scientists to come out and debate all the issues around animal testing. What we wanted was for scientists like Dr Bailey to be able to tell the stories of their own research and to make it very clear what the evidence did and did not support, to avoid any misunderstandings. In this case her results were from a study on mice and had not yet been demonstrated in humans. Our mission is to make science journalism more accurate; avoiding or removing any mention of an animal model from a press release results in journalists reporting new findings as if they apply directly to humans. I remember one study that showed a new treatment led to improvements in hearing when tested on mice. But the university press team removed the reference to mice, resulting in misleading headlines about a breakthrough for the deaf.

I also decided I had to speak out myself – if I was going to ask others to practise what I preached, I needed to show I was willing to do the same. I'm not qualified to speak on animal research from a scientific point of view, but I began writing about the need for more openness. I had pieces published in the *Observer* and *New Scientist*, and got my debut on the *BBC Breakfast* couch. Of course, I wasn't a researcher describing my own use of animals so the risks were lower, but the only messages I got afterwards were supportive (plus one from my mum telling me I needed a haircut). It certainly demonstrated it wasn't inevitable that anyone speaking on this subject in the national news would become a target.

Given the atmosphere around animal research in the UK at the time, it was hard for the SMC to treat the subject in the same way as other issues. While we ran regular press conferences to promote new research findings on GM, MMR, climate change and more, there seemed to be little appetite to run proactive briefings on animal research. In fact, I struggle to remember a single press briefing we ran on animal research that wasn't initiated by us. It had been placed into a whole separate category and I was desperate to change this. To bring the scientific community with us we needed to demonstrate the success of a proactive approach. Without any positive examples, it was easier for the nay-sayers to maintain that the risks of negative stories were too high.

Then I saw my chance. The small community of scientists and organisations who were advocating for animal research transparency had tipped us off in 2003 about the 'annual stats'. Every summer, the Home Office publishes statistics on the numbers and species of animals used in science in the previous calendar year. I was stunned to find such a glorious example of openness. The way in which the data was communicated, however, was less of a cause for celebration. The norm was that the stats were published quietly on the government website, whereupon they were promptly seized upon by animal rights groups who sent them with their own spin to their chosen reporters. It was a huge missed opportunity.

It took three years of meetings, cajoling and persuading to put my plan into action. But finally, in 2006, we held the first SMC animal research stats briefing: a press conference for specialist science journalists with four or five scientists, vets, animal technicians and 3Rs experts available to explain and provide scientific context for any increases or decreases in the figures, as well as to answer media questions about the changes. The result? Media coverage of the statistics was transformed.

Opponents of animal research had routinely used the annual stats to further their agenda, focusing on any numbers that had grown without acknowledging the scientific or medical context behind the rise. For instance, the press release from BUAV on the statistics for 2007 referred to the top-line figure of around three million procedures performed that year, and that 61 per cent of these were carried out without anaesthetic. It didn't mention that these three million procedures included the breeding of one million mice and the taking of blood for research purposes (the animals are bred to have a gene for a specific disease; they do not suffer from the condition). Context is a necessary part of informed understanding of animal research.

The proactive media briefing on the annual stats allowed animal science researchers to communicate the information in a measured and accurate way. Of course, there were some negative headlines: animal research was controversial in the UK and the headlines reflected that. The number of animals used was also large and grew for many years as the life sciences sector in the UK flourished, using animal testing to better understand disease, test the safety of drugs and vaccines, and develop effective new treatments. But the coverage was dominated by quotes and context provided by the scientists. Even in years that saw a large increase in animal research, such as in 2010 when the number of procedures performed on mice rose sharply as part of work towards sequencing the human genome, the press coverage was primarily positive. The *Independent* carried the front-page headline 'The mouse that cured', and went on to cover the story in a double-page spread inside.

However, while we were seeing a gradual change in press coverage when scientists engaged more, we were still dealing with the chilling impact of extremists. In January 2004, while our battle for briefings was still under way, the University of Cambridge announced it was axing its plans to build a new primate research facility after spiralling costs, delays and security concerns. It was seen as a massive win for animal rights protesters, who had opposed the facility on all fronts: enlisting MPs to voice their objections, conducting public opinion polls, threatening to block all roads in the area in repeated protests and even launching a High Court challenge against the government's decision to grant Cambridge permission. After Cambridge had pulled out of its building project, Oxford announced that it too had started work on constructing a major new animal facility. This time, however, things would be different. Then science minister Lord Sainsbury gave the police tough new powers to clamp down on animal rights extremism and funded the huge insurance and security costs for the Oxford building project. Lord Sainsbury was determined that the Oxford lab would be built, and that a message be sent to animal rights activists that they could not close down a legal and legitimate area of scientific endeavour.

Protesters turned their attention to Oxford, where despite these high levels of support from government and the police, the university initially struggled to change its 'head down' strategy. At the height of the protests against the lab in 2004, the BBC's medical correspondent Fergus Walsh called me from a train to Oxford complaining that he had interviews lined up with the activists, but that despite multiple requests, the university had failed to put anyone up for a pro-science interview. The story was set to run on the flagship *Ten O'Clock News*. I managed to track down Professor Tipu Aziz, a leading neuroscientist at Oxford, who used a small number of primates in his ground-breaking research on Parkinson's disease. He agreed to do an interview rather than allow the only voice to be that of the protesters. The next day, a press officer from Oxford emailed to say that Aziz was an inappropriate choice because he was too 'gung ho' in his support for animal research.

Despite the university's caution, we could see that attitudes in both the scientific community and government were shifting. Significantly, support for openness even came from the police. Speaking to the *Financial Times* in 2005, Assistant Chief Constable Anton Setchell, who led the national police campaign against domestic extremism, said: 'This is a lawful, highly regulated activity and I encourage researchers to speak up about it. The extremist groups generate a fear of being victimised that is far greater than the actual likelihood. If people are better informed about animal research, the little support that now exists for extremists' campaigns would be further diluted.' It struck me as remarkable that such a strong statement of support for openness should come from a tactical police unit rather than from the scientific establishment. I spent years sharing the statement with scientists and communications officers who insisted that their security experts were warning them that the threat from animal rights activists was still real. When I explored these warnings, I often discovered that they came from internal security reports about threatened demonstrations on campus. Many of the demonstrations never materialised or involved handfuls of protesters carrying placards.

In 2005, Laurie Pycroft, a sixteen-year-old boy from Oxford became frustrated at the continual presence of animal rights activists in central Oxford. He went into WH Smith, bought some card and a marker pen and made a placard that read 'Support Progress. Support the Oxford Lab', before taking up a stand opposite the

49

activists. News of his defiant one-man protest spread fast, and within weeks Pycroft and a group of university science students had set up a bold new campaign group: Pro-Test. The organisation was not exactly embraced by the university authorities, with members claiming they were not allowed to meet in university buildings. It did, however, capture the imagination of hundreds of Oxford academics who had watched helplessly as the animal rights activists dominated the narrative, and it galvanised those of us who had been fighting a lonely battle. I advised Pro-Test on media strategy, suggesting it appoint press officers and send out regular releases on its own activities and issue comments on developments. I revelled in the group's success, all the more in its boldness and courage – strikingly absent at the highest levels in academia. Tony Blair, then prime minister, penned an opinion piece in the *Sunday Telegraph* that year that expressed support for Pro-Test, and later used a major science speech in Oxford to pay tribute to Pycroft. That a serving prime minister made such a bold statement in support of animal research in a major speech showed how much things were changing.

While the campaign for openness was not generally supported by the scientific establishment, the SMC was never alone. We had a small but steadfast group of allies, from academics and press officers to non-profits, funding bodies, journalists and patients. Some industry bodies, such as the Association of the British Pharmaceutical Industry, openly supported their members' use of animal research and provided support to any who were targeted. Organisations like Understanding Animal Research (UAR – the successor organisation to the Research Defence Society) and the Association of Medical Research Charities had been leading the charge for openness for years before we arrived. There was an intense solidarity among us, forged in the fire of the hostility and fear that this topic stirred up.

I felt particularly encouraged by the bravery of patients who had benefited from research on animals and who chose to speak out on this controversy. One such patient, Mike Robins, had severe Parkinson's disease and was one of the first UK recipients of deep brain stimulation, a ground-breaking technique in which a device placed into the brain helps patients control the extreme tremors that come with the disease. Professor Tipu Aziz was one of the scientists who had developed the treatment and had tested it on monkeys before putting it into human trials.

The two of them made a great double act at public talks and media interviews. Aziz would explain the technique and Robins would then stand up, calmly reach inside his shirt, and turn off the device. The tremors would slowly take hold and after a few agonising minutes, Robins' body would be in the grip of shockingly violent and all-consuming shaking. In one particularly rickety hall, the audience was quite literally shaking with him. Then Robins reached back into his shirt, flicked the switch back on and his body returned to its peaceful state.

I had so much admiration for him. He was battling a nasty disease and probably did not relish the prospect of standing in cold meeting halls defending the need for animal testing to the Women's Institute or animal welfare groups. But he was a great advert for an area of research that so many medical breakthroughs rely on. I was sad to hear from Professor Aziz some years later that Robins had died. I thought of him often over the years when scientists or university comms people declined requests to speak to the media. Like sixteen-year-old Laurie Pycroft, Mike Robins put them to shame.

In 2008, Lord Drayson, a founding board member of the SMC, became science minister under Gordon Brown. Drayson had himself been a target of animal extremists years earlier when he ran a vaccine company called PowderJect. He asked me what he could do as science minister to advance the cause of openness on animal research, and we cooked up the idea of holding a dinner in the Commons, bringing together vice-chancellors and business leaders to encourage a bolder approach. Not everyone responded well to the idea: some vice-chancellors referred to protests on campus as a reason for keeping quiet. This annoyed Phil Willis MP, then chair of the Commons Science and Technology committee. In his broad Yorkshire accent, he said something along the lines of: 'Oh strap on a pair. I had ten people dressed in mouse suits protesting outside my constituency offices last month. I invited them in, made them a pot of tea and debated the issue with them. They were pussycats.' Sometimes however the problem is more about the existing culture within a university, generally set from the top. Some leaders simply want to avoid all possible risk.

Changes in this area came slowly and from different directions. A significant role was played by the UK's science journalists who, like me, were increasingly frustrated at their lack of access to scientists on this issue. Journalists like Rachael Buchanan, Tom Feilden and Fergus Walsh at the BBC and Alok Jha at the *Guardian* had spent years trying to get into animal labs to report this controversial story from the scientists' perspective. While they were always prepared to black out names and disguise buildings to protect researchers, they were losing patience at the disproportionate hurdles placed in their way. When Feilden was finally granted a visit to the empty new animal facility in Oxford, it was on the bizarre condition that he surrender his passport before the visit. Not surprisingly, he declined. These journalists had followed this story for years and could see that some of the precautions were no longer justified by the level of threat from extremists.

The reputational threat of not speaking came into sharp focus for some of the UK's top universities after a story in 2005 by Clive Cookson, long-serving science editor at the *Financial Times*. An advocate for greater transparency on the issue, Cookson was similarly frustrated by the status quo, and we bemoaned the situation over lunch. As the second glass of wine arrived, he shared details of a feature he was planning. The *Financial Times* would send a questionnaire to the UK's top universities asking them a series of questions that would demonstrate their commitment – or lack of it – to transparency. He would write up the results as a feature and push for a leader to go with it calling for more openness. I loved the idea. Those that had been pushing for openness would be able to alert their senior management to the reputational risks of not opening up, while those who had blocked it would feel the heat. Within minutes of Cookson sending out his list of questions, I received my first call from an outraged university head of press, dismayed by what she perceived as irresponsible journalism that would leave her institution and researchers vulnerable to attack. I listened quietly, wondering whether or not to admit to my prior knowledge of and enthusiasm for the piece. She was so cross that I bottled it. After several similar calls had come in, a colleague told me I had to 'fess up'.

One of the calls I remember that day was from an anxious head of communications at a top university who told me that it was halfway through building a new animal research facility in the middle of campus and that she was one of only a handful of people in the university who knew. I suggested it might be time to start telling other academics and students the truth, as someone was bound to find out at some stage, and it was most likely to be the activists first.

The *Financial Times* asked forty-five universities about their policies and whether they encouraged their academics to speak publicly on the issue. Thirty-three universities responded in full, and others gave partial answers. When the feature appeared in October 2005, it had a positive spin. Under the headline 'Openness grows over animal research', Cookson wrote: 'Universities are becoming more open about their animal research programmes, a *Financial Times* survey shows.' He reported that more than half now had a statement on animal research on their websites, adding that many had been added during the previous year. I smiled at the reference to the five statements that had been 'added in the past month', knowing that several had been added in the previous twenty-four hours.

Organising media visits to animal labs became a big part of my strategy of proving that openness did not have to be a risky business. When I had started the job, I had felt queasy about animal research myself and persuaded Andrew Gay, marketing director at Huntingdon Life Sciences (HLS), to let me visit their dog facility. Huntingdon was probably the most beleaguered of all institutions. A contract research company carrying out research for universities and life sciences companies, the organisation had been targeted by the Stop Huntingdon Animal Cruelty (SHAC) campaign since 1999. In February 2001, managing director Brian Cass had been attacked by three men armed with pickaxe handles and CS gas, and in 2010, five SHAC members received prison sentences for threatening HLS staff.

The SHAC campaign had also introduced the concept of secondary targeting. Clients, banks, suppliers and shareholders were all contacted and warned that if they didn't stop working with HLS, they would suffer the consequences. NatWest Bank, for instance, was targeted with a sustained vandalism campaign in which its ATMs and front doors were disabled with superglue. Eventually the only bank that would allow HLS a standard current account was the Bank of England – following an intervention from the government.

Remarkably, HLS's response was to throw open the doors of the lab to journalists, politicians and anyone else keen to find out the truth of what happens in animal labs. My colleague and I spent a day being jumped on and licked by healthy-looking, excitable beagles and talking to vets, scientists and animal technicians who seemed as dedicated to the welfare of the animals as they were to the research projects they were conducting. I had approached the visit nervously but left – as I did every subsequent visit to similar facilities – feeling reassured that what I saw conformed to the highest standards of welfare.

I was convinced that inviting journalists into these facilities was crucial to busting the myths that research animals are routinely mistreated and unnecessarily subjected to severe pain and agonising deaths. Every visit I helped to organise resulted in measured and positive media coverage and it was satisfying to know that people Googling animal research in future would find balanced articles with up-to-date photos of animals housed in good conditions.

One of my favourite examples of a media visit came at the University of Leicester. Like so many universities, Leicester had been upgrading its facilities to the ever-higher standards required by the Home Office regulators, and, like others, it was desperately trying to hide the fact. Just as I'd predicted, the one group of people who knew exactly what was happening were the activists. In 2010 senior scientists working on the new project woke up to a piece in the local paper in which inaccurate claims were reported that the lab would house monkeys and dogs as well as mice and rats. Ather Mirza, then head of communications at the university and a former journalist, was one of a small band of senior communicators who had long been pushing for a more open strategy. Determined to drive home his point that secrecy was not working, Mirza pushed for a bold and proactive media plan, including inviting local and national press to tour the facility. When he asked for our help in the run-up to the centre opening in September 2012,

I offered the chance of a visit to Tom Feilden on BBC Radio 4's *Today* programme who jumped at it.

It's hard to overstate how radical a media strategy this was at the time. Despite the *Financial Times'* report on progress towards openness in 2005, there often wasn't much more than a quiet reference to animal research buried on a university's website. To be out and proud like Leicester was unheard of, as the *Today* programme emphasised in its prime-time slot, presenting the visit to the lab as a major triumph of science over fear. The *Leicester Mercury*, the same paper that had previously reported inaccurate claims about the lab, carried an article on the new facility and a special editorial in which the editor pointed out that the paper's previous coverage had been based on misinformation supplied by activists. Under the title 'Establishing the facts on animal experiment labs', he wrote:

> The University of Leicester has allowed one of our report-ers to see for himself exactly what goes on in the labs. There were no preconditions put on our visit and our reporter was told that he could choose where he wanted to go and could look wherever he chose. The outcome is that we could find no evidence whatsoever of experiments being carried out on dogs or primates. This, combined with the licence conditions and the statements of the university, leads us to believe that no such experiments are carried out. This is not a comment on whether or not vivisection is right – but the argument should be based on fact, not exaggeration and scare tactics.

Today's culture of openness came about thanks to individuals like Ather Mirza at Leicester, and the science journalists who became more critical of secrecy. But it also occurred following a chan-ging of the guard and a new approach from the leaders of the big funding agencies. Professor Mark Walport, who became head of the Wellcome Trust in 2003, was a huge champion of openness, and when the Medical Research Council (MRC) appointed Professor Colin Blakemore to be its head that same year, it was certain that the issue of animal research would no longer be swept under the carpet. Not long after his appointment, I woke to hear Blakemore on the *Today* programme threatening to resign from his new post. A newspaper had found a letter revealing that the professor had been passed over for an honour because of his support for vivisection. Now, here he was live on Radio 4 saying that unless a member of government came out to back him and express the government's support for the use of animals in medical research, he would resign. A few hours later, a government spokesperson issued a statement declaring just such support for animal research and did a round of back-to-back media interviews. I called Carolan Davidge, the MRC's head of media, to congratulate her on her genius media plan. There was a silence on the line before she said: 'Fiona, we knew nothing about it until we heard him on the radio.' Less a brilliantly choreographed PR strategy, more a bold, possibly reckless, instant response from Colin.

In 2012, we got involved in the issue of transportation of animals for research. Given that animal research as a whole was a subject that generally went under the radar, the public naturally knew very little about the way scientists were getting the animals they needed for studies. For years, animal researchers had been telling me that some of the biggest global airlines and shipping companies were no longer transporting animals for research following intimidation from protesters. Every time it was mentioned, I suggested we take the story to the media. That iconic transport companies like British Airways, P&O and Eurotunnel were refusing to accept legitimate and lawful business vital for medical research was shocking, and I felt that the public and policymakers had the right to know about it. Critically the animal breeders and research institutes impacted by the ban could argue that it was adversely affecting animal welfare because it meant longer, more arduous transportation routes for research animals. In turn, that could affect the quality of research because stressed or unhealthy animals could skew the results of experiments. At times, our discussions took a comical turn as lab managers discussed the welfare of animals forced off BA flights to Heathrow onto low-cost airlines into Newcastle. I empathised with the downgraded mice.

Every time I suggested going public, everyone got twitchy. They told me that there were extremely sensitive discussions ongoing with companies and government, and that they had been given assurances that the problem would soon be fixed. But it never happened, even though by this point the animal rights movement was a much less intimidating force. Lord Sainsbury's crackdown had seen most of the ringleaders convicted, and long sentences had acted as a deterrent to supporters whose numbers duly began to drop. Extremism was turning into animal rights activism, which was perfectly legal, much less threatening, and took place mainly online. The upshot was that super-rich, powerful, global companies were often making major decisions in reaction to nothing more than a few tweets. The myth that the situation was 'being resolved' became clear when Stena Line, a major ferry company, announced in early 2012 that it was also pulling out of carrying research animals. I tried my luck again. This time, I got a mandate to go public.

The SMC doesn't normally give 'exclusives' to media outlets, but the scientists involved were too anxious about a widescale media release. With policymakers in mind I approached *The Times* and the *Today* programme. They knew that this was an important and strong story, but they wanted it to be fronted by a big hitter. I suggested Lord Drayson, who had been quiet since losing his job as science minister after Labour's defeat in the 2010 general election, but who still cared passionately about this issue.

With just days to go, everything was going smoothly. *Today* and *The Times* had coordinated closely and chosen a day to run the story. *The Times* was planning a leader to go alongside the breaking news, backing the call for these companies to come back on board. *Today* decided to bid for the serving science minister David Willetts, which of course involved calls to government communications staff. This is where the fun started. Suddenly, senior communications managers in government were very keen to speak to me. In my experience, this is never a good thing. I managed to avoid their calls and emails, but the government instead went to work on spooking the scientists who had agreed to be involved. The message was clear: this story must not happen. The government was on the verge of getting a deal with these airlines and shipping companies and this publicity would undermine years of hard work. Even if it were true that such a deal was close to being agreed – which I did not believe for a minute – this story would be as likely to help seal the deal as destroy it.

The day before the story broke, two senior communications officials from the Department for Business, Innovation and Skills (BIS) turned up at our offices in the Wellcome Trust. In a slightly menacing after-hours meeting, the officials told me that I was putting the future of science at risk and that I would not be forgiven for wrecking the sensitive and fragile behind-the-scenes talks. I thanked them for their time and said it was too late. That night, both Ceri Thomas, editor of *Today* and Simon Pearson, night editor of *The Times*, received calls from BIS officials along similar lines. This was a new situation for me, and I asked them rather fearfully what they had said. 'I told them that their call had guaranteed the story would make the splash,' said Pearson. Thomas had given a similar response. Thank God for a free press.

The next day, *The Times* front page said: 'Medical research is being put at risk because Britain's ferry operators and airlines have capitulated to the demands of animal rights activists not to allow the transportation of mice, rabbits and rats into the country for testing, *The Times* can reveal.' Lord Drayson was quoted as saying: 'By giving in to the protesters, they are inadvertently choking off vital research into some of the most debilitating diseases affecting our society.' Their leader concluded: 'These experiments are a regulated, ethical and integral component of research that saves lives and eradicates disease. They must be not only allowed but enabled to continue.' The rest of the press picked it up. Willetts went on the *Today* programme sounding very cheerful to say his government was bringing the companies together to address it. Depressingly, little has changed since then.

Every couple of years, representatives from organisations involved in animal research are invited into government to hear the results of the polling on public attitudes on the use of animals in scientific research. Even though animal rights activists had dominated the media debate for years, the level of acceptance for animal research among the public remained high, especially for the purposes of medical research – throughout the 2000s and 2010s, on average 70 per cent of the public continued to say they accepted research if it was well regulated and for medical research purposes. But in 2012, the polls showed an unexpected 10 per cent decline in public acceptance. Intriguingly, this came at a time when the extremists had all but disappeared and the sense of a public 'row' had abated. My hypothesis was that the controversy stoked by the extremists had provided a media platform for both sides and that when people were exposed to reasoned debate on the subject, they were generally persuaded of the need to carry out tests on animals – just as my husband had found with his students. Less media interest might be welcome to many in science, but it meant fewer opportunities to remind the public of the necessity of such research.

The time was right for another big push forward – restrictive and secretive policies that made sense in wartime were not needed in peacetime. The aim was to normalise animal research as just another aspect of science communication. At a meeting we held with UAR, the MRC and Wellcome, the idea of a Declaration of Openness on Animal Research was born, partially inspired by Clive Cookson's university survey several years earlier. We spent an agonising but ultimately triumphant summer trying to get the big universities to sign up. While no lies were ever told, we were very keen to let Oxford know that Cambridge was on the verge of signing up, and to point out to each of the Russell Group universities that their absence from the list would be noted. It worked. Not just because of our tactics, but because everything had changed, and people knew it. Secrecy on animal research was no longer justified or acceptable. When we had eighteen top universities on board and published the Declaration in 2012, we approached Professor Sir Mark Walport at Wellcome, who agreed to support and fund UAR to turn the Declaration into a more substantial and binding Concordat on Openness. After wide consultation, including six weeks of engagement with the public, the Concordat was published at an SMC press conference in 2014 with seventy-two signatories. Over a hundred of the UK's top research universities, institutes and companies are now signed up to the Concordat, which commits them to mention animals in their press releases, publish the numbers they use on their websites and be proactive in providing opportunities for the public to find out about research using animals.

The public will probably always have reservations about animal research: such ethical qualms are shared by many of the vets and technicians working with lab animals who devote themselves to improving their welfare, and by scientists who work hard to refine, reduce and replace the use of animals wherever possible. But now, at least, we have publicly available information about this area of science from the research institutes doing it, and not just from the activist groups outside the labs. This has been perhaps the most monumental change in the communication of science in my two decades in the job.

In 2020 and 2021 – for the first time in fourteen years – we decided against holding our annual SMC animal stats press briefing. This was partly because of Covid, but mostly because scientists and their organisations are no longer under the same pressure to hide the role of animal research in what they do or fearful of being found out. The media is now openly reporting on the considerable biomedical advances that scientists have made, thanks in part to research using animals. Briefings in the past few years had attracted only a handful of journalists, compared with the packed-out events of years back. By talking openly about the use of animals in research and establishing it as a normal part of science, we have so successfully defused this once highly controversial topic that journalists now show little to no interest in the subject. As James Randerson, former science editor at the *Guardian*, once said to me: 'Give us full nudity and we lose interest.' Animal research is no longer science's dirty little secret.

3

FIRST THEY CAME FOR THE COMMUNISTS

The bitter row over ME/CFS research

MANY OF US WILL KNOW someone with myalgic encephalo-myelitis (ME) – also referred to as chronic fatigue syndrome (CFS). Perhaps you know several people, given that experts estimate that 250,000 people in the UK suffer from the condition. ME and CFS are not exactly the same – ME is a broad term with no definitive set of symptoms – but they share similarities and are often grouped together as illnesses characterised by long-term fatigue and other symptoms that limit a person's ability to carry out ordinary daily activities. While tiredness is common in many illnesses, it's especially severe in ME/CFS and not relieved by sleep or rest. A characteristic feature is that minimal exertion can produce fatigue and a feeling of unwellness. To the huge frustration of patients, no underlying cause has been found and there is, as yet, no diagnostic test. Many patients refer to developing the illness after serious infections like glandular fever or pneumonia, and some experts think that it may be the end stage of multiple different conditions rather than a single specific one.

I have friends and family members who have suffered from this debilitating condition, and in my thirties I had a small taste of what it might involve. I was on a press trip in what was then Zaire (now the Democratic Republic of the Congo) when President Mobutu carried out his long-standing threat to close the notorious refugee camps in the city of Goma, which had become home to over two million refugees who had fled Rwanda in the aftermath of the genocide. With all scheduled flights suspended, we were stuck in Zaire much longer than planned and I ran out of the multiple antibiotics I take for my cystic fibrosis. Predictably, I got the mother of all chest infections. My first stop when we eventually escaped was at Brompton Hospital, where I was promptly admitted for a two-week course of IV antibiotics. Tests showed that the new infection had gone but I left hospital still feeling unwell. After multiple attempts to return to work, I ended up back at my parents' home in Wales where I lay in bed for weeks on end in a kind of stupor, watching *Dallas* repeats on the television that my dad had moved into my bedroom because a trip downstairs was too exhausting. At various stages, my mum and dad would sit on my bed and ask me if I was depressed. I would insist that I was not and that I had nothing to be depressed about except the bloody illness, often before collapsing into floods of tears. After numerous frustrating and inconclusive visits to different doctors, I started to get some energy back. It was a slow process and while I did get back to work after a few months, I felt generally unwell and horribly tired for around a year.

This experience gave me a tiny insight into just how miserable and isolating ME/CFS can be. I remember pledging to never again complain about my mild cystic fibrosis, with its recognisable symptoms, tried and tested treatments and known timeframes for recovery from infections.

When I started at the SMC, I was interested to meet the

scientists working in the ME/CFS field and talk to them about any exciting advances being made in understanding the causes of the illness and the development of promising new treatments. What I found was a nightmare: a small and beleaguered group of scientists who, despite years of working in their field, were all to various degrees contemplating leaving because of harassment by a group of vocal activists. Since then, our experience of working with these scientists has proved to be a cautionary tale: of what happens when good medical evidence is attacked and misrepresented; of the importance of defending the right of scientists to pursue their chosen field of research even if it comes under attack; of the importance of ensuring that patients and the public can hear about and access evidence even when it is contested by vocal critics; of what happens when a debate becomes so polarised and toxic that campaigners present scientists pursuing valid lines of research as 'waging war' on patients.

Professor Sir Simon Wessely is a pioneering researcher who helped develop the first therapies and NHS clinics for treating ME/CFS. When I first met him, shortly after starting at the SMC, I was appalled to discover that he routinely received death threats and threatening calls, which had forced him to install a panic button in his house and have all of his post checked by police X-ray machines. One website described him as a 'dangerous madman . . . and an obvious sadist'. Another compared him to Nazi death camp doctor Josef Mengele – an especially hurtful accusation since two of Wessely's grandparents were killed in Auschwitz. And, the professor explained to me, he continued to be subject to all of this abuse despite having taken the decision in 2000 to stop his research on ME/CFS.

Shocking as this kind of intimidation is, I discovered that it is far from the only tactic used by the activists: they also make regular formal complaints against individual researchers, which take up huge amounts of time and threaten not only to derail the research itself but to undermine the researchers' integrity and reputation. Such complaints often involve hundreds of Freedom of Information (FOI) requests for emails and data to which the recipients are legally bound to respond – a tactic also employed by activists on animal rights and climate sceptics. By submitting an FOI, anyone in the world can demand to see any written material from UK scientists employed by universities. In one case, scientists undertaking a trial of behavioural treatments for ME/CFS were forced to release 600 pages of ethical committee submissions, all the minutes of their trial management and steering committees, and individual patient data (once anonymised). Participants in this trial had been assured that none of the data collected about them would be publicly released, but an Information Tribunal found against the university, and it was forced to comply. One ME/CFS researcher calculated that dealing with malicious FOI requests of this kind had, at one time, taken up a quarter of his working life.

Many of the scientists involved in ME/CFS research have also been reported by activists to the General Medical Council (GMC) in an attempt to get their medical licences revoked. Speaking to a journalist from the *Observer* in 2019, Professor Michael Sharpe, a specialist in psychological medicine at the University of Oxford, said: 'You find yourself constantly under investigation . . . You can't function like that.'

But what, you might well want to ask, are these activists so upset about? Don't they want to have research conducted into ME/CFS? I can't claim to fully understand their grievances but they appear to object to the fact that many of those involved in researching and caring for ME/CFS patients are psychiatrists, psychologists or behavioural scientists whose work has led to the development of behavioural/psychological treatments such as cognitive behavioural therapy (CBT) and graded exercise therapy

(GET). After many years of having their persistent symptoms dismissed by insensitive doctors and family members, some ME/CFS patients see the predominance of psychiatrists and psychologists working in this field as proof that the medical profession thinks their condition is 'all in the mind' as opposed to a 'real' illness with physical symptoms. Many of these patients also believe that the focus on behavioural therapies for ME/CFS has discouraged other types of scientist from conducting research into the illness, with the result that possible biological causes and alternative treatments remain unknown. Some argue that ME/CFS will only be taken seriously when psychiatrists are off the scene, whilst others openly state that their goal is to discredit and drive these scientists out.

Some experts I have spoken to feel that the objections voiced by ME/CFS activists draw a strangely anomalous dividing line between the practice of psychological and physical research into the illness. Arguing that doctors increasingly acknowledge that there is a complex interplay between mental and physical health, they have called for a new way of talking about the nature of illness that avoids the kind of outdated dualism that suggests it has to be either physical (and real) or mental (and imagined). Modern medicine, they say, is focusing increasingly on treating the health of the person as a whole. So in the case of ME/CFS, they believe it is wrong to reject the possibility that physical symptoms can be treated with psychological approaches, and also that such objections inadvertently risk reinforcing the stigma around mental illness.

One thing all sides agree on is that many ME/CFS patients have had a miserable time. In the 1980s and 1990s, as awareness of the illness grew, it was often referred to as 'yuppie flu' – a derogatory term referring to the seemingly high number of affluent city dwellers brought down by the illness. Patients have long reported being dismissed as malingerers by GPs, or have argued that their physical symptoms were too quickly written off as depression or some other psychiatric illness. Although not specifically about ME/CFS, a damning 2001 academic survey of GPs showed that 64 per cent thought that patients with 'medically unexplained problems' had a psychiatric illness and 84 per cent thought they had 'personality problems'. The irony here is that initially, unlike other specialists, it was psychiatrists and psychologists who chose to step forward to acknowledge the suffering of these patients and conduct research to develop treatments. My assessment has always been that ME/CFS patients have indeed been ill-served by medicine, but that their frustration and anger has found the wrong target.

One of the stories I worked on that highlighted several of the challenges was the October 2009 publication of a paper in the respected US journal *Science* showing that a retrovirus typically found in mice called XMRV had been found in more than two thirds of ME/CFS patients. We hadn't seen the embargoed study, so the first we heard about the story was waking up to the news headlines. The *Independent* had it as the splash, with a headline reading: 'Has science found the cause of ME? Breakthrough offers hope to millions of sufferers around the world'. This seemed like the holy grail for ME/CFS. It appeared to show that the illness was indeed caused by a virus. Better still, it was a recognised virus for which there were already drug treatments available. As news media across the world announced that a cause and potential cure for ME/CFS had been found, the SMC was left scrabbling for third-party comments – too late to engage very effectively with the news story.

I was annoyed that we had more or less missed the boat but I was even more upset when we did speak to scientists and found that they were a lot less excited about the study than the news reporters were. The number of patients in the study was small, and researchers could not understand how this attempt to identify a viral cause of ME/CFS had proved so decisive when previous attempts had come to nothing. The consensus was that this was potentially significant, but the results would need to be replicated by other labs. Unfortunately, few of these cautionary comments made it into the excitable headlines, and by the end of that day patients were ordering antiviral drugs off the internet and a test for XMRV which just happened to be marketed by the same lab. I remember Sarah Boseley, the *Guardian*'s veteran health editor, telling me how she had argued with her news desk to keep it off the front page. She had covered this issue for years and felt that this single study finding had a smell of 'too good to be true' about it. She was right.

The first UK lab to attempt replication was at Imperial College London where virologist Professor Myra McClure set up a similar experiment. When her paper was published in January 2010, she approached the SMC to host a media briefing. We bit her hand off. Having missed the original story, we were keen to engage with a study that could potentially confirm such a significant finding. Unfortunately for us, and for patients who set so much store by it, McClure and her colleagues sat in the SMC and explained to the journalists that her team could not replicate the findings. In fact, they found no trace of XMRV in any of the patients. Pressed by reporters, she speculated that the dramatically different findings might be because the samples in the original study had been contaminated. As other labs around the world also failed to find the virus, more questions were raised about the original paper and in December 2011 it was retracted by the journal, a drastic last resort for studies that have been found to have serious flaws. Aside from the specifics of ME/CFS, this story was a great example of why journalists should resist the temptation to oversell single studies. As I've mentioned before, one of my oft-repeated maxims is 'extraordinary claims need extraordinary evidence' and this was one without the other. But the excitement said everything about a media and patient community desperate for a breakthrough in this area.

Dashed hopes have been a painful recurrent feature of ME/CFS research. But so has the hostile reaction to inconvenient findings. Professor McClure was a virologist and not in any way a ME/CFS researcher. But soon after the SMC briefing, she asked to be removed from any lists associated with the illness. She had been subjected to a barrage of online abuse – one activist had written to her repeatedly saying that he was imagining watching her drown, and she had to cancel a planned visit to the USA after police advised her that death threats from US ME militants were 'credible'. McClure later told a BBC journalist about her experience. 'It really was quite staggeringly shocking, and this was all from patients who seemed to think that I had some vested interest in not finding this virus,' she said. 'I couldn't understand, and still can't to this day, what the logic of that was. Any virologist wants to find a new virus.' McClure made it clear that, in response, she had decided not to do any further research in this area.

In 2011, we were approached by the lead author of a new clinical trial set up to compare different treatments for ME/CFS – known as the PACE trial. Professor Peter White from Queen Mary's University of London knew the risks inherent in any media launch about ME/CFS and had reservations about even holding a press briefing. Initially, and naively, we thought White was exaggerating the extent of any potential controversy – surely such a briefing would be the best way to ensure that journalists were offered an accurate account of the findings. The trial was funded by the Medical Research Council (MRC), the Department of Health and the Department for Work and Pensions, and was due to be published in the *Lancet*, both reassuring signs that this was good-quality medical research. Having convinced White to go ahead with the briefing, our next step was to persuade all the other relevant press officers to get involved too. All of them knew more than we did about the potential for controversy surrounding the results of the trial and were nervous, but for that reason they felt a press briefing where the researchers had proper time to describe the details of the trial and highlight its limitations was a good idea. The next few weeks involved intense preparation, including a full dress rehearsal with SMC press officers playing the role of journalists asking tough questions.

I suspect clinical trials similar to PACE, in which different treatments are tested against each other to see which ones work better, are generally uncontroversial in other classes of disease. The PACE trial was designed to compare three of the treatments for ME/CFS commonly offered to patients. A total of 641 patients with ME/CFS were recruited from six clinics across the country and divided into four groups. Everyone was given specialist medical care as standard. One group received no further care, but each of the other three was given a different additional treatment: adaptive pacing therapy (APT), where patients adapt their lives to live better within the limits of their condition; CBT, which aims to help patients explore ways to understand their illness and cope actively; and GET, where patients are encouraged to gradually increase the time they are physically active.

The trial found that, one year on, patients offered either CBT or GET (as well as specialist medical care) experienced more improvement in relation to their levels of fatigue and physical function than those offered either APT (with specialist medical care) or specialist medical care alone, and additionally found that all four treatments were equally safe. These findings were consistent with several previous trials, and the National Institute for Health and Care Excellence (NICE) was already recommending these treatments for anyone with the condition. What was significant about PACE in comparison with other trials was that it was the largest study of its kind. None of the scientists involved were claiming that any of the treatments involved were a cure-all, and they were clear that CBT and GET could offer only moderate benefits on average, but until something better was discovered these were the best options.

The press conference went smoothly. We had reassured the authors that the science and health reporters present would ask tough but well-considered questions and report the study fairly, and they did. And for the first time, I witnessed just how good these scientists were at communicating their findings. The journalists knew enough about the past history of this illness to raise questions about the nature of ME/CFS – terms like 'yuppie flu' and 'all in the mind' came up – but Professors Michael Sharpe and Trudie Chalder, who led the trial with Professor White, answered their questions clearly and skilfully. I was to hear these particular answers from ME/CFS researchers many, many times over the years. That ME/CFS is a genuine illness that can cause severe disability and distress. That ME/CFS is not 'all in the mind' and that they reject any description of any illness in those reductionist terms. That physical and psychological factors are important in all illnesses. That CBT and GET are medical treatments that this, and previous trials, had indicated could help some patients. That in the absence of a definitive explanation for this illness, the responsibility of medical researchers in the field is to do further research, test treatments and gather robust evidence about what does and does not work.

Despite all of our preparation, the PACE trial went on to become a lightning rod for activists' anger. It has variously been attacked as 'scientific and financial fraud', 'a piece of crap' and 'one of the biggest medical scandals of the twenty-first century'. Formal complaints have been lodged with the *Lancet* (which has consistently refused to retract the study), the MRC, and more recently the Health Research Authority (HRA), which was set up in 2011 to set the standards for clinical trials in the UK, and there are constant claims that the trial is 'discredited'. All the PACE trial doctors who led centres were reported to the GMC, responsible for the regulation of doctors in the UK, which subsequently determined there was no case to investigate in all instances. There have even been debates in parliament about the PACE trial, with at least one MP using parliamentary privilege to allege that the trial was fraudulent.

No clinical trial is perfect. Most contain flaws of some kind, but I can think of no other clinical trial that has been subject to such intense and sustained scrutiny and criticism. Hundreds of thousands of words have been written alleging shortcomings. Some of the main ones revolve around which patients were included, how the outcome was measured, and a lack of access to the trial data. PACE, however, has been scrutinised repeatedly by various scientific bodies. Despite huge pressure, the MRC and the *Lancet* have stood by the trial. More recently, Professor Sir Jonathan Montgomery, then head of the HRA, investigated the trial after he was questioned about it by MPs in January 2018 while giving evidence to a House of Commons Science and Technology Committee inquiry on research integrity. His report, published in early 2019, not only described PACE as a good trial but praised it for being ahead of its time in its transparency and ethical standards: 'We commend the investigators of PACE for recognising the importance of transparency by acting on good-practice recommendations for publication on protocols and the statistical analysis plan even though they are not regulatory requirements. These are practices that we would want to encourage and this openness has enabled proper scientific debate.' Rarely has a piece of medical research been so vilified or so vindicated.

The press conference for the PACE trial went well, but working closely on it with the authors, funders and journal was a baptism of fire for us. I was shocked by the levels of anxiety we found among those involved with the trial, and again by the reaction of scientists when we tried to do our 'roundup' of third-party opinion about it. By 2011, these roundups were a routine part of our work, with scientists generally enjoying the opportunity to see and comment on new findings in their field before publication. But we were learning fast that normal rules didn't apply here. Most of those we approached refused to comment. Some were honest. They had seen what had happened to colleagues who engaged publicly on this issue and were not prepared to risk becoming targets themselves. Others had direct experience of commenting on ME/CFS and had pledged never to do so again. Some ruled themselves out for reasons that we knew would not have deterred them on any other issue. Some independent experts cited conflicts of interest because they had some distant connection with the PACE trial – a frustrating experience for us. Others became uncharacteristically modest about their expertise. One way or another, we learnt the hard way that most scientists do not want to talk to the press about ME/CFS.

This reluctance struck at the heart of our mission. The SMC exists to encourage researchers to speak out on the messy, controversial issues in science so that the public and patients have access to the best evidence and analysis. Here was an illness which some estimate affects one per cent of the UK population in some way, but scientists were scared to talk about it. What to do?

In March 2011, we decided to bring together some of the scientists affected by this harassment to see if collectively we could come up with a solution. We were joined by some ex-police officers who had set up an organisation called Support4Rs to advise scientists targeted by animal research extremists, and by

GMC experts who were dealing with multiple complaints against ME/CFS doctors. At the meeting, we raised the prospect of the researchers going public about their harassment. We had only learnt the extent to which they were being silenced after witnessing it at close quarters – the wider scientific community and the general public were completely unaware of what was happening. Based on our experience of working with similarly beleaguered animal researchers, we hoped that raising awareness about the harassment of scientists in the ME/CFS field might galvanise wider support for them from the scientific community and science journalists.

Initially, the scientists at the sharp end were wary. They worried that going public might provoke the activists and invite more abuse. We put the idea on the back burner, but were convinced as a team that this situation was showing no signs of improving and that the right kind of media spotlight could bring about change. We also had a strong sense that things could not get much worse. By this point, Professor Sir Simon Wessely had left ME/CFS research and was studying the effects of armed combat on the mental health of soldiers. His reference to feeling safer travelling to war zones in Iraq and Afghanistan than researching ME/CFS often got a laugh from audiences. But he was not joking.

In the end, our hand was forced. Tom Feilden, science editor on BBC Radio 4's *Today* programme, had picked up on the climate of fear around this issue. He brought it to the attention of the programme's then editor Ceri Thomas who was shocked and became equally keen to run some kind of piece about it. Feilden approached us about it and we discussed what such a piece might look like. We asked him to give us some time and said we would talk to the scientists to try to convince them to participate. He agreed, but made it clear he would start looking into it and that *Today* would cover the story regardless. We went back to

Professors Wessely, Sharpe, Chalder and others with a more pressing case. The story might run with or without them. We believed that engaging with the programme was the right thing to do and promised to be with them every step of the way.

In the event, the *Today* programme, so often dominated by politics, devoted a large amount of its time to the story one day in July 2011. Feilden did a live piece at 06:30, with Wessely following live at 07:30. The 08:10 slot, usually reserved for the big political interview of the day, was a lengthy pre-recorded package which included Wessely again, as well as Professor Myra McClure and Dr Esther Crawley, a paediatrician from the University of Bristol specialising in ME/CFS. Professor Sir Mark Walport, Head of the Wellcome Trust, and Dr Charles Shepherd, medical adviser to the ME Association, did live interviews as well. It was huge.

The next few days were remarkable. Professor Wessely and Dr Crawley did back-to-back interviews, many of which were long, detailed and sympathetic. These are scientists who have dedicated their careers to improving the lives of sufferers. The general reaction was shock that a group of respected scientists had been subject to an unpleasant campaign of such vitriol that some had felt they had to walk away from this field of research. My hope was that we would look back on this moment as the one when the medical research community realised the need to mount a more public defence of colleagues working in controversial areas. Sadly, that was not to be.

Scientists were not the only targets of abuse. Science journalists who have reported on ME/CFS studies have also found themselves vilified online and subject to aggressive complaints. When journalist Michael Hanlon told me he was planning a feature on ME/CFS for the *Sunday Times* magazine in May 2013, I tried to prepare him for the likely reaction. Opening the piece, he wrote: 'The story of ME activism is probably not one you will have heard much about, even though it is just as controversial as vivisection. Because not only do doctors who work in the field get a lot of grief, so does any journalist who covers the story. I was told by more than one colleague that I was mad to even think about writing about it.' Privately, several journalists have confessed to me that they want to avoid the subject where possible, given the level of criticism and complaint that inevitably follows.

It's important to emphasise that it is only a tiny number of patients whose frustrations tip them into the targeting and harassment of researchers. They claim to represent all ME/CFS patients, but they do not. Outside this minority, some patients are frustrated by the lack of research into the condition and report poor outcomes from the treatments recommended by the NHS, and some deeply resent any implication that their illness is 'all in the mind'. Both groups are well represented by several patient charities, including the ME Association which lobbies for more research funding and better treatments. There are also plenty of patients who have a more positive experience of services, and credit doctors with helping them manage their symptoms or even recover. They tend to stay off social media and avoid what they see as a toxic debate. The varying attitudes of these different patients are perfectly legitimate, and it would be beneficial to everyone for these discussions to happen openly and freely. But the chilling effects of the actions of a handful of activists have undermined any productive conversations. In the end it is both science and patients who lose out in that atmosphere.

***

The SMC is sometimes accused of being too close to a small group of experts, on this and other subjects, and some feel that ME/CFS has become monopolised in the media by scientists with a particular perspective. That may be fair comment, but the irony is that the numbers of experts is small because scientists from different fields working on the condition mostly want to stay out of the media. The SMC has a range of experts on this subject on its database, including researchers looking exclusively at biological aspects of the disease, but, despite our best efforts, most scientists in the field are reluctant to talk to journalists or speak at our press briefings. The result is that most media requests for interview still end up going to the same handful of scientists. Professor Sir Simon Wessely generally starts by refusing, but often makes the fatal mistake of saying, 'Come back to me if you really can't find anyone else.' I've lost count of the number of times I have had to call him back and heard that sigh of resignation as he reluctantly agrees to the interview. When asked, Dr Esther Crawley says she does it on behalf of the patients in her clinic who believe in her team and the treatments they offer and want her to be their voice. And Professors Michael Sharpe and Trudie Chalder say they do media because it's crucial to hold the line in defending legitimate research from illegitimate attack. Mostly, I think they all end up doing it because they know no one else will.

Our interaction with the media on ME/CFS is qualitatively different from other issues we cover. Journalists reporting contentious subjects like statins, antidepressants or e-cigarettes often come to us asking open-ended questions and are keen to produce balanced reports. But on this subject, much of the media interest starts from the 'row' and many journalists have decided their angle before they start. Rather than being asked about the evidence base for understanding and treating ME/CFS, experts are often asked to defend their research from a familiar list of criticisms. Such bad-faith journalism serves no one.

One example of this sticks with me. In January 2018 a journalist writing for *Nature*, one of the world's most respected science journals, sent email messages to the authors of the PACE paper requesting an interview. She explained that she had been working on her piece for some time, but had just been asked by her editor to submit it quickly and to include comments from them. The authors were given twenty-four hours' notice to agree a time for interview. It was clear that contacting the UK's primary ME/CFS researchers was an afterthought in an article that had been months in the making. The scientists were worried that the piece would just be the latest in a long line setting up a false dichotomy between exciting new molecular biology research and 'discredited' psychological approaches. Despite my best efforts, I couldn't persuade them to speak to the reporter at such short notice, though they offered to do so in a more reasonable time frame. When the piece came out, PACE was referred to alongside the XMRV trial in a short paragraph about 'controversial research' that had 'marred' the reputation of the research field. The piece claimed that a new group of medics was finally listening to patients after years in which doctors had dismissed their symptoms. I helped the PACE authors to write a response – partly because they felt demoralised by yet another misinterpretation of their work, and partly because it was important to put their objections on record. In it, they made a significant point about the way in which objections to their research have been shaped by misperceptions or assumptions:

> It is regrettable that some patients and others link behavioural treatments with dismissal of a person's condition, when in fact these therapies can be beneficial ... In our view, there is no place for stigmatising any avenue of research or therapy that might help us to improve the lives of people with this long-term debilitating illness.

One BBC programme about school-age patients with ME/CFS, and arguably not really about PACE at all, involved a presenter grilling the authors for an hour over criticisms of their work. The programme was an interesting and valid investigation, but once again it seemed a journalist had come to the story with a pre-conceived angle. I persuaded the researchers to engage but they were even more unhappy when they discovered that the presenter was a journalist who had worked on an episode of *Panorama* covering a similar subject, about which the BBC had previously upheld a complaint. I was in awe of the scientists for the patient and open answers they continued to give. Most scientists who have worked on a clinical trial will never answer media questions about it. Some working on trials with big public interest may do media work for a day or two when it's published, but then move on and never do further media work on that particular trial. These authors were still answering critically framed questions on their trial six years after it was published, some after moving into different areas of research completely.

Every time we had media enquiries like these, we tried to involve spokespeople from the many universities, funding agencies, journals and medical research organisations that were linked to PACE and its authors. Not just to lift the burden from the small group who were under the cosh, but because we felt it was important for the public and patients to hear that the wider medical research community was involved with and supportive of the trial. We spoke to organisations including the MRC, the HRA, the *Lancet* and Cochrane – a world-renowned international network formed to summarise and publish the best evidence from medical research – asking them to speak out about the evidence base for current treatments. They told us they believed in the quality of the medical research available, and broadly rejected the criticisms circulating on social media and among patient activists. A statistician who worked on PACE told me that she uses it in her training programme as an example of a good clinical trial. Very occasionally, we persuaded them to speak to the media or issue a statement, most notably when Professor Fiona Watt, the new executive chair of the MRC, sent a letter to *The Times* defending PACE in August 2018. In it, Watt said:

> As funders of the PACE trial, we reject the view that the scientific evidence provided by the trial for using CBT and managed exercise in the treatment of CFS (also known as ME) was unsound ... It is important that researchers are not discouraged from working on the disease because of concerns that they could be subject to the level of hostility that PACE researchers have experienced. Medical research can only flourish when there is mutual respect between all parties.

Mostly, however, we failed spectacularly. The list of reasons given for refusing our requests was long and became all too familiar. It was not a priority for them. They were no longer funding those researchers. They felt it was better for A. N. Other to comment. They were now funding biological research. They were too close to the research. They were too far from the research. Organisations that were otherwise beating a path to our door to speak out on a wide range of subjects did not want to speak on this issue. Some were brutally honest and told us they were deliberately avoiding speaking in the media because they had neither the heart nor the institutional capacity to deal with the inevitable backlash. And who could blame them? But that didn't mean it didn't matter. It did. For future controversies as much as for this one.

While the medical research community collectively walked away from doing media work on this issue, campaigners against PACE continued to lobby organisations to withdraw support from the trial and its findings. In October 2018, Reuters health and science correspondent Kate Kelland broke the news that Cochrane was planning to withdraw its systematic review of GET for ME/CFS after complaints from patients and campaigners. The authors of the original review objected, and after protracted and tense discussions, a compromise was reached: the authors revised their review to emphasise the limitations of the available evidence and the publisher agreed to keep the review in the Cochrane Library. As an attempt to chart a course through these perilous waters, it was not hugely successful. Campaigners were now opposed to the revised review, while researchers were concerned about the potential implications of the decision. Speaking to Reuters when the story first broke, Professor Sir Colin Blakemore, the neuroscientist who had suffered so much abuse from animal rights extremists, warned that the withdrawal decision set a worrying precedent for scientific evidence and was 'a departure from the principle that has always guided Cochrane reviews – that they should be based on scientific and clinical evidence . . . but not influenced by unsubstantiated views or commercial pressures'.

In September 2017, NICE announced a review of its guidance on the treatment of ME/CFS as a response to a sustained campaign by activists. In November 2020, the organisation published its draft guidance, which banned GET and downgraded CBT. These recommendations were a significant change to the previous 2007 guideline, which had recommended both treatments on the grounds that 'currently these are the interventions for which there is the clearest research evidence of benefit'. The new draft recommendations were also made in the face of even greater evidence for the efficacy and safety of these treatments than had been available to the previous guideline committee, including the biggest trial of these treatments ever published. Campaigners welcomed the draft, with many celebrating what they saw as the end of harmful treatments being offered on the NHS. On 18 August

2021, NICE was due to publish the final version that medical professionals would have to adhere to, unless there were specific reasons not to do so in the case of an individual patient. But in the run-up to the announcement, the media reported that three members of the committee had resigned because they felt unable to sign up to the final guideline. All three were NHS healthcare professionals who led or worked at major NHS ME/CFS services.

In the following days, it emerged that several medical bodies including four Royal Colleges – of General Practitioners, Paediatrics and Child Health, Physicians, and Psychiatrists – had lobbied NICE after discovering that many of the detailed points they had made in their responses to the consultation had not made it into the final draft. Their main argument was that the review of the evidence base seemed to have been manipulated to fix the evidence against CBT and GET, with even a Cochrane review supporting GET being sidelined. It was reported that the NHS had also made strong representations expressing serious reservations about withdrawing treatments from patients without any alternatives to offer. In an extraordinary move on the eve of expected publication, NICE pulled the plug on the guidelines at the eleventh hour, issuing a press release saying: 'Because of issues raised during the pre-publication period with the final guideline, we need to take time to consider next steps. We will hold conversations with professional and patient stakeholder groups to do this.'

We gathered reactions from experts to news of the delay. Dr Alastair Miller, a consultant physician in internal medicine and infectious diseases, has been caring for patients with ME/CFS since the early 1990s. He acknowledged the ongoing controversy, but pointed out that CBT and GET remain the only evidence-based treatment approaches to ME/CFS and withdrawing them would leave many patients with nothing. He expressed his disappointment at the decision and his concern that it had been 'based more on political pressure than good science'. By contrast, Professor Chris Ponting, principal investigator at the MRC human genetics unit at the University of Edinburgh, said the guidelines should receive support from professionals and patients, pointing out that 'consensus decisions were taken by the panel' and that they were rigorously developed by NICE.

What struck me in the responses was that both sides said that NICE had bypassed its standard processes and buckled to external pressures. Many of the scientists and professional bodies felt that NICE had agreed to review its guideline and made the changes about GET and CBT because of pressure from patient groups, while the patient groups identified the last-minute lobbying from the NHS and Royal Colleges as the reason the guideline was not published as planned. NICE did eventually publish its guideline on 10 November 2021 after a round-table meeting in which a variety of different views was heard. The final version was very similar to the draft and confirmed that GET would no longer be a recommended treatment on the NHS, and CBT could only be recommended as a symptom-management tool.

I have no idea what lessons NICE will take from this tale of woe, but I think it's fair to say that its well-deserved international reputation for neutral and objective assessment of the evidence has been dealt a blow in some science circles. One friend who worked in the NICE media team before this story said that while she enjoyed the job, it could sometimes be a little boring because NICE decisions must be standardised and formulaic, leaving little scope for creative press-release writing. I suspect public trust in NICE derives precisely from that reputation for impartial assessment of the evidence in determining what works best. It's certainly why I trust it.

NICE and Cochrane are not alone in coming under pressure from patient activists. Every organisation that has anything to do with medical research on ME/CFS has experienced intense and often unreasonable lobbying from campaigners. Some have had moments of bravery where they have issued statements or done the occasional interview. But mostly they try to keep their heads down, avoid the issue and hope against hope that it will go away.

By 2016, we had to acknowledge that our attempts in 2011 to raise media awareness of the treatment of researchers in this field had not succeeded in galvanising a united front from the scientific community. The 'strength in numbers' principle that finally threw a protective blanket around those individuals who had been targeted by animal rights activists had not worked with ME/CFS. If anything, things were getting worse.

Not surprisingly, this toxic environment has continued to have a chilling effect on those actively involved in research and means that the wider public and patients with the illness are not hearing from experts involved in the research and care of patients. I have had many moments of despair on this issue over the years, but one I particularly remember was when we learnt that a scientist who had authored an update on PACE had asked the *Lancet* media team not to publicise the findings because of the potential backlash. Not wanting to do media interviews is one thing. Actively suggesting that new research findings are not put into the public domain because of fear is another. Surely anyone who believes in the scientific endeavour can see that this situation is untenable.

My colleagues and I feel that there is a wider principle at stake here. If a group of scientists and a body of evidence can be silenced or discredited in this way, what's to stop other activists doing the same with other findings they don't like? The answer is that there is nothing we can do to stop them trying – but we can, as a scientific community, think about how we can better defend researchers, evidence and the scientific process from such attacks.

The SMC is not in the business of championing one area of research or backing a particular approach. We have worked hard to run briefings on new approaches to ME/CFS and would love to see funders supporting new and promising directions. We're in touch with scientists carrying out biological research into the area, including genome study DecodeME and a biobank of ME/CFS patient samples collected for researchers' use. We watch the USA with interest and hope that increased funding for ME/CFS by the National Institutes of Health there will start to deliver fresh promise. We are optimistic too that some good may come from the parallels noticed between ME/CFS and what has been termed long Covid. Coverage of the latter condition in the media has been sympathetic, which may draw new scientists and funding into a field of science that could bring benefits for ME/CFS patients. But championing new research avenues should not mean demonising existing research. It seems likely that ME/CFS is a collection of different symptoms and causes in need of a multi-faceted approach. We need different groups of researchers looking at different aspects. But we also need an atmosphere in which different research is discussed and debated openly without fear – and without the sense that one avenue of research or treatment somehow undermines or challenges another. Robust critique of evidence is part of the scientific process. Vexatious and aggressive attacks that aim to close down an area of research and drive scientists out of their jobs will ultimately damage all avenues of investigation and put scientists off entering this important field. If that happens, patients will be the ultimate losers.

In 2019, Reuters published a major feature on ME/CFS by Kate Kelland. It showed how the campaign against scientists researching behavioural therapies had resulted in a reduction in the numbers of scientists working on ME/CFS and the amount of research being published. It concluded that the activists may have inadvertently achieved the opposite of their goal. By attempting to discredit one area of research, they had in effect discouraged scientists from other areas entering the field altogether. Dr Lillebeth Larun, a researcher at the Norwegian Institute of Public Health who has worked on Cochrane Reviews of treatments, told Kelland: 'Attempts to limit, undermine or manipulate evidence-based results, pressure or intimidate researchers into or away from any given conclusions, will ... only lead to those researchers choosing to work in other areas and reduce the resources dedicated to providing the help patients so desperately need.'

In all my years working closely with scientists on this issue, I have never heard them speak about ME/CFS patients with anything other than sincere empathy and compassion. Some continue to see patients in their clinical practice, and I have met patients who credit them with their recovery. There is no doubt that ME/CFS patients have been treated badly by some GPs and neurologists, and by sections of the press. That is not acceptable and we should all rage against it – but that rage should not be targeted at scientists who have devoted their research and clinical lives to understanding and treating this disease. Despite the hostilities between them, I genuinely believe patient groups and the scientists we work with want the same thing – for ME/CFS to be taken seriously, and for patients to have access to a better scientific understanding of their illness and improved treatments. I really hope I will live to see an end to the war on this issue, because I am convinced that no one benefits from it.

Thankfully the situation with ME/CFS is extraordinary and rare. But the principles involved are not. My real worry is that the collective failure of the medical research establishment to step into this row to publicly support the scientists, defend a body of evidence and argue that we need all kinds of research to tackle this devastating illness will pave the way for the same thing to happen in other areas of science. Substitute the words ME/CFS in this chapter with other contested issues like vaccines, climate change, autism, statins and you can see the dangers. We need scientists to feel able to discuss their disagreements in the media free from fear. Sadly, this story feels like the cautionary tale of this book. The one where everybody loses.

4

HYPE, HOPE AND HYBRIDS

The battle for research on human–animal hybrids

I KNEW SOMETHING was amiss when I saw the way Dr Evan Harris was working the room at the SMC's 2006 Christmas party, leaving groups of scientists, journalists and press officers looking animated and concerned. A former medical doctor, Harris was at that time the Liberal Democrat MP for Oxford West and Abingdon – one of a tiny number of politicians at Westminster who understood and cared about science. He was a dynamic member of the House of Commons Science and Technology Select Committee and his obsessional eye for detail could be infuriating – I came to dread him producing some huge wedge of committee papers in a bar to show me one minute point that he was cross about. But everyone I knew in science loved having such a dedicated champion of evidence and reason in Westminster, and when I woke up after the 2010 election to learn that he had lost his seat, I felt bereft.

The news he was breaking at the Christmas party was that, buried in the small print of the government's revised Human Fertilisation and Embryology (HFE) Bill, published that day, was a move to ban research on human–animal hybrid embryos. Tony Blair's government was responding to perceived public revulsion at the prospect of researchers using such embryos to better understand and treat disease; what we saw was a major test for our belief that scientists could change public opinion by engaging with it more boldly. It would prove a key moment in the changing culture of science communication.

The notion of creating human–animal hybrids emerged from research using embryonic stem cells – a type of blank cell able to generate all the other specialised cells required for our bodies to function. By harnessing the unique properties of stem cells, scientists were able to 'grow' other types of cell and study them to understand how diseases develop and which drug treatments might be effective. Stem cells sourced from adults are more limited in their ability to produce other types of cell, so scientists preferred to extract embryonic stem cells from eggs that had been fertilised at an IVF clinic but never implanted in a woman's uterus. But this process too had its drawbacks: fertilised eggs were in short supply and they only allowed scientists to study human cells in general rather than those of a specific patient.

It was to address both of these issues that scientists then developed an approach called 'therapeutic cloning'. This involved taking an unfertilised human egg, extracting its nucleus (which contains the cell's genetic material), and replacing it with a nucleus extracted from the cell of an individual patient. This then allowed them to create stem cells genetically specific to a particular patient, which in turn could be used to grow all the specialised cells that might be relevant to understanding or treating that specific individual's illness.

However, even though unfertilised human eggs can be more widely available than fertilised ones, their supply was still insufficient to meet the demands of this hugely promising research.

And this is what prompted some experts to propose the use of animal eggs to create a therapeutically cloned human–animal hybrid. Science journalist Alok Jha provided this explanation of the process:

> In making the hybrid, the animal egg is hollowed of all genetic information and replaced with the nucleus of a human cell. The resulting cell is then induced to divide and eventually becomes an early-stage embryo. Genetically the hybrid is 99.5 per cent human ... the stem cells exist inside this early-stage embryo, ready to be extracted for research.

Before the idea of human–animal hybrids entered the conversation, one of my early jobs at the SMC had been to ensure that journalists understood the distinction between therapeutic cloning and human reproductive cloning, which has been explicitly banned in the UK since 2001. One of the biggest stories we had dealt with in our earliest years was the claim made by maverick IVF doctors Dr Severino Antinori and Dr Panos Zavos that they had cloned a human. Back then, such announcements tended to attract headlines despite a total lack of evidence to substantiate them. I will never forget the Christmas holiday in 2002 spent gathering responses to fresh claims of the birth of a human clone made by the Raëlian Church, a previously unheard-of US sect. Such assertions were being announced in plush hotel rooms rather than in scientific journals or conferences, in briefings heavy on PR but light on evidence. Amid growing anger from mainstream stem cell scientists, in January 2004 I organised an open letter to the media calling on journalists to think again about reporting new claims of cloning humans without evidence. The signatories feared that the disproportionate coverage these stories were given conveyed the impression that fertility scientists in general were racing to clone the first human, a concern regularly raised by my Irish Catholic mother who had not been delighted when I left a job at a Catholic aid agency to enter the world of science. In those early days, she called me after every high-profile human-cloning claim to complain loudly about these scientists who think they can play God, while I tried my best to explain that the mainstream experts I was working with were united in their opposition to this work.

Therapeutic cloning for research purposes, on the other hand, was very much on the agenda, and we were already talking to scientists keen to win public and political support for this endeavour. One of those was Professor Ian Wilmut, a research group leader at the Roslin Institute at the University of Edinburgh, famous for having cloned Dolly the sheep. In February 2005, I flew to Edinburgh to run a press briefing at which Ian explained to journalists why he was teaming up to work on a project to generate patient-related stem cells through cloning, working with Professor Chris Shaw, head of Clinical Neuroscience at King's College London, Professor Richard Anderson, professor of Clinical Reproductive Science at Edinburgh, and Dr Paul de Sousa, senior lecturer in the Centre for Regenerative Medicine at Edinburgh.

It was soon after this that I learned for the first time that scientists were exploring the possibility of using animal eggs instead of human ones. I was told about it by Professor Robin Lovell-Badge, head of developmental genetics at the Medical Research Council's (MRC) National Institute for Medical Research, who said that he had visited a lab in Shanghai where scientists claimed to have successfully generated embryonic stem cell lines from rabbit and cow eggs. Keen that we share this information with journalists, I organised a background briefing in August 2005 with Lovell-Badge and his colleagues Professor Anne McLaren, from Cambridge, and Dr Stephen Minger, from King's College London.

That press briefing was an important milestone in our attempts to change the culture of science communication. There was as yet no new study nor a funding announcement, and no rising public concern about the use of human–animal hybrid embryos. So why rock the boat? Why risk generating scary tabloid headlines sooner than was absolutely necessary? The answer was clear to me. These scientists were seriously considering seeking regulatory approval to use these embryos. Explaining their reasoning publicly was the right thing to do. It demonstrated that researchers were open about their work, willing to answer media questions and address any public concerns. It meant journalists heard it first from the scientists themselves, rather than the 'pro-life' lobby or one of the single-issue groups opposed to embryo research; and equally importantly, that the British public therefore heard it first from science journalists, who would report the facts accurately. Exactly what had not happened with GM crops in the 1990s.

As it turned out, the media could not resist some scary head-lines. But that was to be expected: most of the time, journalists don't write their own headlines, a situation that often leads to a significant gap between what the headline suggests and what the actual article says. Here, the explanations beneath the headlines were measured and accurate. A key group of science journalists now understood the processes of cloning and deriving patient-related stem cell lines, and why scientists were struggling to get the number of cell lines they needed from the limited supply of human eggs left over from IVF. The scientists had given a clear explanation of why using animal eggs would allow this research to go ahead without subjecting women to intrusive, potentially risky egg collection.

Above all, the briefing was a proof of concept for a new, pro-active approach to controversial subjects. The British public had learned about human–animal hybrid embryos from scientists talking to science journalists early on before a controversy had even begun. Some press officers might call it controlling the narrative. I called it openness.

Six months later, that background briefing would stand us in good stead. Scientists interested in therapeutic cloning in the UK had been open about their interest in the techniques of South Korean scientist Professor Hwang Woo-suk. When the professor published a paper in May 2005 in *Science* describing the first successful patient-derived cell lines, we ran a briefing for the journal, hosted in the UK because of the toxic atmosphere surrounding stem cell research in the USA. It attracted journalists from all over the world. Seeing a group of burly Korean security men standing guard at our doors was almost as exciting as having world-class stem cell researchers in our office. But that Christmas a scandal broke when it was alleged that some of the data in the South Korean lab had been fabricated. We issued a response, but it was clear that the UK's science journalists needed to speak to scientists directly. By this stage, Professor Alison Murdoch from Newcastle University had become the first UK scientist to follow in Professor Hwang Woo-suk's footsteps, publishing a paper following his protocols to derive patient-related cells from a cloned human embryo. The press understandably wanted to know where any falsified data from South Korea would leave UK scientists and this whole field of research.

I hastily assembled a panel for the first day back in the office after the Christmas break and brought together as many of the experts as I could. At that press briefing, Professor Chris Shaw was specifically asked where he and Professor Ian Wilmut would get their supply of eggs. Shaw replied that they were about to apply to the Human Fertilisation and Embryology Authority (HFEA) to use human–animal hybrids. The cat (or in this case rabbit or cow) was well and truly out of the bag and the coverage was prominent in the next day's papers. 'Clone team want to grow human cells in rabbit eggs', said the *Daily Mail*, while the writers at the red tops had fun with their headlines, with the *Daily Mirror* running the story under 'Eggs grow into bunnymen'.

Despite some sensationalism in the headlines, I was delighted. The media coverage was another example of scientists telling this story in their own words. There was a principle here. To risk-averse PR executives, this briefing could have been seen to have back-fired – exactly the type of situation that convinced most press officers in the past to avoid proactive media work that could go wrong. But what had actually gone wrong? The scientists had shared their plans openly and responded to the intense media interest by carefully explaining what the science involved and how it might help them treat currently incurable diseases such as Parkinson's, spinal-cord injury and some forms of blindness. A story like this one, involving medical, legal and ethical issues, is inevitably controversial and messy, and the press coverage will always reflect that. Keeping your head below the parapet and hoping it somehow all passes off without criticism is simply unrealistic and ultimately counterproductive.

During 2006, stories about human–animal hybrid embryos returned to the news on several occasions as different groups of scientists applied to the fertility regulator for licences to use them and we prepared for the regulator's decisions. It was at this point that Evan Harris dropped his Christmas party bombshell: research on human–animal hybrid embryos would be banned in the updated HFE Bill.

The next couple of weeks were a whirlwind of activity. From what we could work out, the Department of Health had decided to ban the use of human–animal hybrids due to little more than the response to a hastily arranged public consultation. Scientists we worked with were wary of the ways in which such consultations could be hijacked by pressure groups. Some of those opposed to stem cell research were driven by religious concerns about scientists 'playing God', and many were active in pro-life anti-abortion groups. Others felt that stem cell research might start by focusing on incurable diseases but that it would inevitably lead to more sinister efforts to clone human beings or create 'designer babies'.

There is a fine line between communicating science accurately and campaigning for a particular stance or outcome, and sometimes that line can get blurry. The *Fields of Gold* saga (see Chapter 1) had left me wary of straying into campaigning territory. But listening to the scientists and patient charities affected by the proposed ban on hybrid embryo research left us convinced that something important was at stake here. This was not curiosity-driven research being carried out by vainglorious scientists intent on playing God. The purpose behind this research was to better understand illnesses such as muscular dystrophy, dementia and motor neurone disease (MND) – conditions for which there were no cures, or even effective treatments. To ban an avenue that offered researchers better ways of studying these diseases and testing new drugs was not trivial. As Professor Shaw put it when explaining why he had become involved in this research: 'I had been working in an MND clinic for more than two decades. During that time, many drug trials had come and gone without any real breakthrough. My patients were dying, usually within two years of diagnosis.'

I set up a press officers group, and Sarah Norcross at the Progress Educational Trust arranged a wider group involving the key scientists and policy officers. With little or no precedent for this kind of co-ordinated response in the science community, we put together a kind of war council to look at ways to overturn this proposed ban. The SMC's role in this was obviously to work with the media, and the first thing to do was consider how to bring the issue to their attention. At that point no news outlet had picked up on the ban: it was hidden at the back of a White Paper packed full of interesting and important updates on fertility treatment, which were of huge public interest. I argued that we should not say anything until January: my feeling has always been that once Christmas party season gets under way, politicians and the public pay less serious attention to news. We decided to run a briefing on the first day back in the office in January 2007, bringing key scientists together to challenge the ban and make their case for why they needed human–animal embryos for their research.

The timing of the briefing went down badly with Rachael Buchanan, a senior medical producer at the BBC and one of the best science journalists I know. Buchanan had been at our Christmas party and knew scientists like Professor Robin Lovell-Badge and Dr Stephen Minger, whose team had also put in an application to use hybrid embryos, as well as I did. She had woken up after our Christmas party with a hangover and a determination to break the story. We had woken up with the same hangover, but the opposite conclusion – the story had to wait. By the time Rachael called Lovell-Badge and Minger asking for interviews, I had already persuaded them to hold off talking to journalists until the January briefing. Buchanan was understand-ably livid, and I remember us shouting at each other on the phone as I attempted some last-minute Christmas shopping in TK Maxx. She argued that it was not our story to embargo, and we had no right to tell these scientists not to do an interview with the BBC. She pointed out her excellent track record on covering this issue, and forcefully told me that I was completely out of order. She was completely right. But so was I. This was not just another story. It was the start of an unprecedented fightback against a government ban on legitimate research.

To have maximum impact on policymakers and the public, we needed to make sure that all the news outlets would run the story on the same day at the same time. An embargo was the only way to do it. Embargoes are always controversial, and never more so than artificially created ones like this. The knowledge that the government had proposed a ban on hybrids was already in the public domain. But scientists could decide how and when to let people know their response. There would be other occasions where I would urge scientists to give a journalist an exclusive story, but this was not one of them. Not for the last time, we had to admit that as close as we sometimes get, given our often complementary roles, there will always be a tension between journalists and press officers. Luckily, Buchanan forgave us and was sitting in the front row at that January press conference.

The embargo on the briefing lifted at midnight and we woke up to the story dominating the *Today* programme on Radio 4, and generally all over the news media. 'Medicine faces ban on rabbit–human embryos', said the front page of *The Times*, with a standfirst that read, 'Move hits hopes of Alzheimer's sufferers', and that ministers were 'caving in to religious groups'. 'Hybrid embryo ban "would cost patients' lives"', ran the headline in the *Daily Telegraph* and 'Scientists denounce plans to outlaw "chimera" embryo experiments' was how the *Daily Mail* ran the story. The articles beneath the shouty headlines were glorious, full of quotes from the scientists on the panel and clear 'explainers' from the science journalists. The story was now being informed by science, not ideology. Many newspapers added extra reports to the main news with fact boxes and infographics explaining the technique. Some papers carried opinion pieces from science journalists like Mark Henderson in *The Times* arguing against the ban. In an op-ed under the title 'Ministers have been spooked by "frankenbunny" headlines', Henderson noted the uncharacteristic media strategy:

'It's not often that British scientists involved in embryo research club together to berate ministers for overzealous regulation that has not been properly thought through.'

Over the next eighteen months, hardly a week went by without a development and part of our media strategy was to ensure that each one was an opportunity to get scientists into the mix. We ran press briefings or issued responses when the HFEA announced that it would be unable to grant licences given the proposed ban; when it launched its public consultation; when it concluded its public consultation; when the Academy of Medical Sciences (AMS) published its report on inter-species embryos; when the Science and Technology Select Committee published its report recommending the technique be allowed, and so on. We worked with press officers from the MRC, the AMS, the Wellcome Trust, the Parkinson's Disease Society (now Parkinson's UK) and more, all assembling at our offices for a coordination meeting every few weeks, usually at the end of the day to allow for a glass of wine or three. Perhaps most powerful of all in terms of shifting public opinion was the involvement of the Association of Medical Research Charities (AMRC) and the Genetic Interest Group (now Genetic Alliance UK): between them, they represented the views of over two hundred patient-research charities from the Alzheimer's Research Trust (now Alzheimer's Research UK) to the Muscular Dystrophy Campaign (now Muscular Dystrophy UK). They demonstrated that patients were strongly in favour of allowing scientists to pursue this research and – even better – were able to offer journalists compelling case studies for their reports.

The opposition to legalising research on hybrid embryos had come primarily from the Catholic Church and a couple of campaign groups with a long track record of opposing embryo research, cloning and 'designer babies': Comment on Reproductive Ethics (CORE) and Human Genetics Alert. Led by Josephine

Quintavalle and Dr David King respectively, these were small organisations with little by way of public backing, yet their names appeared in much of the media coverage about this issue over the two years that the story ran. Very occasionally, a journalist would admit that they were struggling to get a reaction comment because these go-to 'antis' were not answering their phones.

As MPs prepared to debate the HFE Bill in May, the issue of hybrids rose higher up the political and media agenda, and politicians and church leaders began speaking out. I have a funny relationship with the Catholic Church. I was brought up in an Irish Catholic family and, unlike friends from similar backgrounds, had never turned against the Church. I credited my education at St Richard Gwyn Catholic High School with making me an independent critical thinker with a strong moral compass. Before moving to the SMC, I had spent seven very happy years at CAFOD, a Catholic overseas aid agency. Though I was no longer a practising Catholic, I was what Clare Short, former Labour min-ister, once called an 'ethnic Catholic'. I had a soft spot for the Church's teaching on social justice and liberation theology, but despite having been taken on pro-life marches with my mum when I was a child, my earliest disagreements with the Church had been on pretty much everything the hierarchy said on contraception, abortion, IVF and embryo research.

So it had been a relief to me that the Catholic Church seemed to be largely staying out of the debate on hybrids. All that changed on a Sunday in January 2008. My mum was staying with us, so I took her to Mass in our local parish in Wood Green. To my dismay, the priest read out a letter from the Catholic Bishops' Conference of England and Wales about the HFE Bill including a section on the creation of hybrids – a process it inaccurately described as mixing a human egg and animal sperm to create half-human, half-animal embryos. The letter described such research as 'a radical violation of human dignity' and asked parishioners to lobby their MPs to vote against the bill. I left my mum and young son in the church pew and went outside to call Dr Minger, Professor Shaw and other scientists to brief them on what had been said and to ask for their responses. I was hopping mad about such a misleading and inaccurate presentation of the facts, and was determined to encourage the scientists to respond. Within hours of the Bishops' statement being read out in every Catholic church in the UK, the scientists were doing the rounds of radio studios and talking to print journalists, pointing out the multiple inaccuracies in the statement. Dr Lyle Armstrong, a Newcastle University researcher whose team was to be granted permission to create hybrids that same month but faced the prospect of an almost immediate ban on doing so, pointed out: 'The aim of our experiments is to discover ways to make stem cells to treat human diseases, not to give birth to some abnormal chimera. Even if this were possible, it has no scientific or moral justification and is in any case strictly prohibited by the legislation.' As Professor Shaw put it, the 'radical violation' here was of the truth.

The Church upped the ante again over Easter 2008. Just weeks before the Commons vote, Cardinal Keith O'Brien, the leader of the Catholic Church in Scotland, used his Easter Sunday sermon to condemn the creation of hybrid embryos as a 'monstrous attack on human rights'. He went on to describe the experiments as of 'Frankenstein proportions' and 'grotesque' and 'hideous'. The sermon was issued to the press in advance, and ran in full on the BBC website on Good Friday. The press lapped up the strong language and the story dominated the news for the rest of the Easter weekend. Dr Minger and Professor Lovell-Badge spent their Easter break bolting from interview to interview as a result.

On the Saturday, Jim Devine, Labour MP for Livingstone and a practising Catholic who supported the bill, appeared on the *Today* programme offering to set up talks between the Catholic Church and researchers. I hastily called Tom Feilden and asked if the MP was still in the studio. He had just left, so I sent Feilden chasing after him down the corridor. The subsequent conversation I had with Devine led to a public debate between the Church and the scientists. This unprecedented event was hosted by the Wellcome Trust and sponsored by Professor Colin Blakemore and Archbishop Peter Smith. The BBC made a special one-hour radio programme on the debate, which was broadcast on BBC Radio 4. After the event, Blakemore and Smith reflected on the benefits of such an event in providing a space for each side to listen and understand each other better. It didn't resolve the dispute of course, but Smith described it as providing 'a model for a national bio-ethics committee' to discuss such complex issues, while Blakemore added that 'polarisation of the debate on stem cells serves no one'.

The other thing I did that Easter weekend was lobby the AMRC to bring forward the publication of a joint letter it was working on that showed that all 150 medical research charities it represented wanted this research to be allowed to progress. The letter had been planned for some time but was not quite ready. I argued that the news vacuum over Easter was the perfect time to get it out to the press, and it would be the perfect response to the much publicised Catholic Church attack. The AMRC's press and policy manager was cautious, worried that rushing it would look too much like it was PR driven. But she agreed, and I sent it to the press under embargo until Easter Monday. It got huge coverage. Fergus Walsh's report for the BBC's *Six O'Clock News*, repeated on the *Ten O'Clock News*, was striking. As he spoke to camera, a screen behind him scrolled through the long list of names of patient research charities backing the call, from familiar ones like Cancer Research UK and the British Heart Foundation, to smaller ones for diseases most people have never heard of. His segment finished before the full list of 150 could be shown. It made for powerful TV.

My memory of the weeks running up to the Commons debate is of a frenetic, intense and slightly bonkers period. A hard-core group of scientists, press officers and policy wonks spent as much time in the Palace of Westminster as we did in our offices, hanging out with sympathetic MPs including Dr Evan Harris and Dawn Primarolo, a health minister at the time. But there is one less pleasant memory. Devine had also been keeping up the momentum, booking meeting rooms and connecting policy officers and scientists with ministers. At one stage, he asked me for a favour, explaining that the staff in his constituency office were great practical jokers. Reluctantly and ill-advisedly, I agreed to help with a prank of his own, and at his suggestion duly left a message on his office answer machine pretending to be a reporter enquiring about expenses claims. When his office manager called me back, she sounded so worried that I confessed at once that Devine had put me up to it and had assured me it was a joke. I thought no more about it but was horrified when, over two years later, Devine went before an employment tribunal accused of unfair dismissal, with this incident part of the evidence against him. I was mortified. There followed a terse meeting with the then SMC chair Dr Peter Cotgreave. Having satisfied himself that I had no real connection to the case, he told me to never do anything so idiotic again. I didn't. Devine was later given a sixteen-month prison sentence and barred from seeking re-election following the 2009 MP expenses scandal.

As the countdown to the Commons vote on the HFE Bill began, so the scale of media activity increased. Against my better instincts I was persuaded to run a press briefing specifically for political journalists. The issue of who covers science stories was a hot topic at that time: many people felt that the coverage of GM crops and the MMR vaccine had gone wrong because they had generally been covered by reporters who weren't science journalists. There seemed to be a tendency in newsrooms to believe that science stories could only ever fall into three categories: dinosaurs, space, or something quirky to fill the 'and finally' slot. As a result, if a scientific controversy started drawing in politicians and commentators, it was no longer thought of as a science story but often handed instead to political hacks or general news reporters. But by 2008 this was happening less and less. Editors were increasingly deferring to their specialist reporters, and some told us the change had come about because they realised they had got this wrong with their coverage of the MMR vaccine. However, I could not convince the policy officers from Wellcome, MRC and elsewhere that the specialists would be left to cover the story this time. They were certain that, as we moved towards a Commons vote, editors were bound to pass this science story to their political reporters, and that we needed to brief them to ensure that the coverage was accurate.

I therefore planned a press briefing in the Commons aimed at political and lobby journalists as well as the specialists, and persuaded the scientists to brief a whole new set of journalists to ensure that the measured and accurate reporting we had got so far would continue up to the day of the vote itself. I spent days trying desperately to reach political reporters and lobby hacks to let them know that they would have an opportunity to be briefed by the main scientists involved in a story they were about to be asked to cover. It was funny, then, to open the briefing room door only to see a row of familiar faces in the front row. There were no political reporters there at all – just the same science and health specialists to whom the scientists had been speaking for years. It was further evidence for my case that science reporters were enjoying a newfound status in the UK's newsrooms. Neither the journalists nor their editors had any intention of passing this story to political reporters who would be unfamiliar with the science or the main characters involved.

On the evening of 19 May 2008, MPs voted with a huge majority to pass the HFE Bill. By that time the lobbying from the research community had ensured the bill now included the right of scientists to use 'human admixed embryos', a wider category including both human–animal hybrid embryos and genetically altered human embryos, for research purposes. Prime Minister Gordon Brown and Secretary of State for Health Alan Johnson had indicated that they were supportive of it and the HFEA had already begun to give out licences. Almost every national newspaper had run editorials backing the scientists and the Catholic Church's intervention had completely failed to convince the public that these scientists were doing something monstrous. It was a victory for science but also a huge vindication for scientists choosing to speak up, a point not lost on several journalists. Mark Henderson at *The Times* wrote a piece crediting the change of culture in science for bringing about the kind of debate that had previously been missing on embryo research.

I later heard Dr Lisa Jardine, the well-known historian who would go on to chair the HFEA, telling a 400-strong audience at a lecture theatre that she had been ashamed of the British press during the debate on hybrids. I did not know Lisa at the time but was so upset that I wrote to her to suggest that her judgement was grossly unfair. Yes, the headlines had often been sensational, even ridiculous, with terms like 'designer babies' and 'Frankenstein' peppered all over the coverage, along with images of giant-sized rabbits or humans with cows' heads. (One piece from the *Sun* showed a picture of a woman's body with a cow's head next to the headline 'I'm a bit of a cow'.) But the actual articles were measured and accurate, often using fact boxes and simple diagrams that explained the science better than any scientists had managed to do. And that's the key point. The mass media had demonstrated just how well they can report messy and controversial science to a huge audience when scientists help them to do so. From that 2005 background briefing we ran explaining why there might be interest in using animal eggs, through the move to ban this approach, and ultimately to its public and political backing in May 2008, science journalists had stayed with the story. It was one hell of a ride. But the media had played a key role, the public were well informed, and science had emerged victorious.

Not everyone was pleased, of course. At a retrospective event on the bill in March 2009, Josephine Quintavalle from CORE accused the SMC and the journalists we worked with of dominating the media debate to the exclusion of other voices. It was a message repeated from a very different source when journalism academic Dr Andy Williams from Cardiff University published a study showing that media coverage of the issue had favoured pro-hybrid sources. I wasn't sure whether to feel defensive about these criticisms or to take a bow. The SMC had been set up because debates about similarly controversial topics had often been heavily skewed against mainstream scientists by media-savvy campaign groups, influential religious organisations and maverick scientists. Our founders had wanted to change that, and to see scientists take their rightful place in these debates – explaining the science and challenging misinformation peddled by campaign groups. It felt as though we now stood accused of being too successful.

Our critics were also wrong in assuming that we were trying to close down debate. In fact, the opposite was true. We can't prevent controversy or sensationalism, but we can use them as a golden opportunity to encourage scientists to embrace debate and engage with the public. I have always baulked in meetings where press officers talked about keeping critics out of the media. I had no desire to drive the Catholic Church out of the debate about embryo research. If the scientists ultimately dominated this debate, it was because, when faced with a more level playing field than had previously been the case, the media and the public found their arguments more compelling and persuasive.

What of that thin line between communication and campaigning? I freely admit that this kind of media work is as close as we have come to campaigning for science. When faced with a ban on an important area of research, the science community had little choice but to turn into campaigners for policy change. We are part of that community. Opposition to the government's plan to ban hybrid research was rooted in a strong consensus among medical researchers; had that not been the case, we would have had a different strategy. We regularly object to and do not want to generate the kind of 'false balance' sometimes seen in the media, where two opposing positions are presented as equally valid regardless of evidence.

Over the last ten years or more, we've seen similar media debates over attempts to allow women with mitochondrial disease to have healthy babies through mitochondrial DNA transfer (known in the press as 'babies with three parents') and discussion of the genome editing of embryos that could eventually allow us to cut out faulty genes that see terrible diseases passed from one generation to the next. We now assume and expect that science and health journalists in the UK will report these issues accurately and responsibly – a far cry from the days, less than twenty years ago, when debates were dominated by sensational headlines screaming about designer babies and scientists playing God.

US reporter Charles Sabine has watched the efforts of UK scientists in stem cell research with intense interest, both professionally and personally. His father had Huntington's disease, a horrible disorder which usually begins to appear in middle age and results in jerky and involuntary movements, changes in behaviour and a progressive descent into dementia. Huntington's is a hereditary single-gene disorder, so Charles knew he had a 50 per cent chance of getting it too. Because there is no effective cure or treatment, a positive diagnosis is of limited value and many people in Charles's position choose not to be tested. But Charles had taken the test in 2005 and was found to be positive. When Cardinal O'Brien launched his attack on stem cell research in 2008, Charles had already witnessed his father die a terrible death and was watching his older brother in the relatively early throes of what would be a fifteen-year battle with the illness. He ended up doing loads of media interviews about the proposed bill, offering a patient's perspective.

In an essay about his experience of campaigning on this issue, Charles spoke about the way anti-science voices had dominated the media debate on embryo research in the early part of the twenty-first century: 'I had been noting how, since the start of the stem cell debate at the beginning of the decade, the naysayers and doom merchants had set the agenda. This I realised had left the scientists, the infantry of the advance, on the back foot and forced to react from the position of social outcast.' Few would recognise that description of scientists today.

The issue of hybrid embryos, with its mass of legal, ethical, moral and religious issues, was always likely to be controversial. This story had all the potential to spark a public outcry that might have derailed any hope of developing stem cell research to study human disease. But the proactive approach from the scientific community meant that this time that did not happen. Issues like human animal embryos, mitochondrial DNA transfer and genome editing will always lend themselves to alarmist headlines. But this story proved that such media rows don't have to result in the public turning their back on these new advances. When scientists embrace controversy, go on the front foot and patiently explain their work to journalists, they can bring the public and politicians with them.

5

THE SACKING OF DAVID NUTT

The politicisation of science

IT TOOK ME SEVERAL YEARS to realise the full extent of the government's control over the media work done by scientists whose public funding means that they are in some way connected to the corridors of power. I wish I had remained in blissful ignorance for longer because, once noticed, this quickly became one of the biggest frustrations of my working life. Our remit at the SMC is to remove the barriers that prevent scientists from engaging with the media. Well, one of the biggest barriers in the UK right now is the knock-on effect of centralised government communications encroaching into the media work of publicly funded scientists.

It's a complex issue and, as broadcasters might say, other interpretations are available. Here you are only getting my view, that of a press officer heavily biased in favour of separating science communication from government communication. But I believe there is a fundamental principle at stake. Science communication – like science itself – should be free from politicisation, and separated from a system that is set up primarily to communicate the priorities of the prime minister and departmental ministers. If there are controls and restrictions on scientists talking to the media and the general public, then we do not have sufficient transparency.

I heard the news that Professor David Nutt had been sacked as the government's 'drug tsar' in late October 2009, while I was driving my son Declan to the cinema. It was half term and, so far, my plans to spend time with him had been largely thwarted by events at work. I was determined to have one day off and arranged the cinema trip. It was Declan who took the call from a colleague and relayed the news as we were on the busy North Circular. My initial shouty expletives were followed by instructions to Declan to call some other names in my phone to break the news and tell them I would be in touch soon. This quickly got confusing: at one point, Declan informed Mark Henderson from *The Times* that Mark Henderson had been sacked. No one could ever accuse me of being a slick PR operator. I didn't abandon the cinema trip, but I had to sneak out of the film for a while to work with my colleagues to gather responses from across the scientific community.

Professor Nutt is one of the UK's leading neuropsycho-pharmacologists, specialising in research on drugs that affect the brain. In January 2008, he was appointed by then Home Secretary Jacqui Smith as chair of the Advisory Council on the Misuse of Drugs (ACMD) – or 'drugs tsar' as the role is referred to more popularly. The news of his sacking less than two years later wasn't entirely a shock. Earlier in 2009, Nutt had been very publicly taken to task by Smith after doing media work on a study he had published that suggested the risks involved in taking ecstasy were statistically no more significant than those of horse riding. Smith had taken to the airwaves to rebuke her own drugs adviser and demand he apologise to the families of young people who had died after taking ecstasy, saying: 'I'm sure most people would simply not accept the link that he makes up in his article between horse riding and illegal drug taking.'

Good scientists do not make things up, of course. And Professor Nutt is a very good scientist, one who for some years had been speaking in the media about his scientific work on evidence-based approaches to drug classification. He cited research in support of his conclusions that illicit drugs should be classified according to the actual evidence of the harm they cause, pointing out that alcohol and tobacco caused more harm than LSD, ecstasy and cannabis.

Smith's objection to Nutt was not based on a critique of his methods or the reliability of his conclusions. Her problem, it seemed, was that his findings were inconvenient to government policy and deeply unpopular with sections of the public and press.

After a day of headlines reporting the home secretary's call for him to say sorry to bereaved parents, Nutt issued an apology. I was dismayed at his decision to do that. He was not a politician who had made a gaffe and needed to apologise to save his career. He was an eminent scientist discussing his research findings in the pages of a learned scientific journal. I called him that night to ask why he had agreed to apologise. He explained that he had done so because he felt he could do more to achieve an evidence-based drugs policy by staying on as chair of the ACMD.

Ultimately, his apology was not enough. Fast forward eight months and Alan Johnson was now home secretary, but the tension between minister and adviser remained. Things came to a head thanks to a scientific lecture that Nutt had given comparing the relative harms of drugs, including cannabis and alcohol. The lecture itself had been delivered months earlier at King's College London and the evidence he drew on had been previously published in peer-reviewed journals, most notably in a 2007 paper in the *Lancet* about scales of harms from different drugs including cannabis, alcohol, tobacco and harder drugs such as cocaine and heroin. As chair of ACMD, Nutt had to submit such talks to officials at the Home Office and, on that occasion, they had given him the all-clear. But in October 2009 his speech was then published as a review article by the event organisers and picked up in the media. It was amid the resulting furore that the home secretary sacked him.

If Nutt had been ready to bend to government after Smith's earlier warning, he was in no mood to go quietly now that he had actually been removed from his role. Like other scientists before and since, he learned the hard way that if you fall out of favour with government, the government press officers who had previously been your official press team (in this case within the Home Office) are more likely to be briefing against you than setting up your interviews.

This was exactly the kind of story the SMC was expected to work on. It was contested science in the headlines and it highlighted the way government was prepared to misuse science when it didn't fit with its preferred policies. It also moved the debate about the relative harms of drug use from the pages of learned scientific journals into the news headlines, providing an opportunity for scientists in this field to engage the wider public. Not many research studies on drug harms make it on to the front pages.

Within hours of his sacking, Nutt was doing back-to-back interviews defending himself and his research. With demand high, I set up a press conference for journalists to hear directly from him. I remember an electric atmosphere as the UK's science and health hacks squeezed into the room. The professor was running late and arrived breathless and agitated, with no time for a pre-briefing chat or a calming cup of tea. As I led him past the assembled journalists to the top table, he asked them angrily, 'Who is here from the *Daily Mail*?' while waving around a copy of an excoriating column published that day by Melanie Phillips, a notorious anti-drugs campaigner. Throughout the briefing, Nutt referred to several things that the *Mail* piece had got wrong. The *Daily Mail* reporter present that day was David Derbyshire, a well-respected science journalist who had recently moved to the *Mail* from the *Daily Telegraph*. I tried several times to point out to Nutt that Phillips was a columnist, not a science reporter. But it was too early for nuance. Afterwards, I asked Derbyshire if he was OK about being chastised so publicly for something he didn't write. He smiled wryly and said: 'Well, Fiona – he's not a man troubled by self-doubt, is he?' It's an expression the SMC has since adopted to describe a number of eminent scientists we encounter.

Outraged by Nutt's sacking, two members of the ACMD resigned in protest immediately. The row was growing in the media and scientists anxious about the wider implications of the sacking looked towards Government Chief Scientific Adviser Professor John Beddington and Science Minister Lord Drayson with the expectation that they would speak out. Drayson had been out of the country when the sacking took place, but once back he came under pressure to speak publicly. I had a call from him asking if I could be in his office in the Commons within ten minutes. I could, and I was. My memory is of walking into a room occupied by about half a dozen young men in suits, all seemingly less than half my age and none too happy to see Drayson consulting a nobody like me. I worked out they were special advisers (SPADs) from Alan Johnson's department, Number 10 and the Cabinet Office. Addressing me as if they were not there, Drayson explained that they were in his office to suggest to him that if he went public with any criticism of Johnson's action, he would damage his standing in government and he might find it difficult to get ministerial backing for some of the changes he wanted to make as science minister. I said what I assumed he knew I would say (and no doubt what he was thinking himself): that scientists and the public expected to hear from him; and that there were broader principles in this case about independent scientific advisers being free to publish research that might not align with government policy or public opinion.

By the time I arrived back at the office, Mark Henderson at *The Times* had tweeted that Drayson had given him an interview expressing sympathy for Nutt and criticising Johnson for not consulting his colleagues in government. When the piece appeared in *The Times*, a government insider was quoted as saying: 'At the time Alan Johnson took this difficult decision . . . Lord Drayson was on holiday in Japan playing with motorcars, which would not have made it easy for the home secretary to run it all by him.' Ouch!

Over the subsequent days and weeks, Professor Nutt became a household name, winning the PR battle with government by making himself easily available to the media and making his case with passion and clarity. Months later, I attended a public meeting where the professor was speaking to a packed audience of over five hundred. Nutt's sacking had given him some celebrity, and I think he decided to use a bad situation to good effect. If the government could not stomach him on the inside, he would take his crusade for evidence-based drugs policy to the wider public.

Not everyone in science sided with Nutt. Some felt that his dismissal was inevitable because he refused to accept that evidence should inform policymaking, rather than dictate it. As one person put it to me, politicians must speak in languages other than science. As it happens, I tend to agree with those who quote Churchill's dictum that scientific advice to governments should be 'on tap but not on top'. I am persuaded that democratically elected governments are entitled to decide drugs policy (or indeed any policy) on the basis of a range of views, including those from the police, drugs workers, the electorate, and yes, even the *Daily Mail*. But accepting that politicians have every right not to follow the science was not a justification for removing a scientific adviser because he spoke out about evidence that was at odds with government policy. As Mark Henderson argued in his excellent book *The Geek Manifesto: Why Science Matters*, the key to disputes between government and its scientific advisers is transparency. Politicians have every right to reject scientific advice, but they need to publish it and explain why they have come to a different conclusion.

I was curious as to why some leading voices in science were so privately hostile to Nutt's approach. Years later, I was advised by a good friend inside government that the SMC needed to decide between wanting influence over government policy and criticising it in public – because you can't have both. He explained that 'trusted friend' status is generally granted to those who air their concerns in private.

I hate this notion. Why can't government have a relationship with constructive critics who speak out about how government policy should change? And why should debates of real public importance only take place behind closed doors? I suspect the public debate on drugs can cope with an outspoken scientist who believes that science should be 'on top'; arguably, we would all benefit from an intelligent airing of different views. I also noted ruefully that most of those who were critical of Nutt's approach were reluctant to provide us with comments. If our roundups of scientific reaction looked one-sided on this particular issue, it was partly because his critics within science were not prepared to enter the fray.

The sacking of an independent scientific adviser raised broader questions about the relationship between scientific advisory committees (SACs) and government. I have always been impressed by the way government departments invite independent scientists to feed into government policy through a large number of SACs on subjects ranging from air pollution to pesticides. But very soon after I entered the science world it became clear that while these groups of scientists are often fiercely independent from government in their operational work and advice, they have little or no autonomy when it comes to the communication of that advice. Mostly, it is handed over to government departmental press teams – whose primary task is to support the priorities of their ministers – to share with the media and the wider public.

Determined to get something good out of the Nutt saga, I joined forces with a small group that included Tracey Brown, the director of Sense About Science, Dr Evan Harris, then the Liberal Democrat science spokesman, and Professor Colin Blakemore, the immediate past head of the Medical Research Council (MRC). Together, we co-ordinated the drafting of a new set of principles 'for the treatment of independent scientific advice', and got twenty-eight high-profile scientists – including current and former chairs of independent expert advisory committees – to endorse them.

Professor Beddington and Lord Drayson then announced a review of the principles around independent scientific advice, which led to some clauses being added into a revised version of the government's code of practice for SACs like the one Nutt had chaired. The thing I lobbied for the most in the consultation was for SACs to be encouraged to communicate their work separately from the government and allowed to use their own independent science press officers. But what appeared in the revised advice was a watered-down version that made this separation the exception rather than the rule:

> While it is often appropriate for an SAC to use its sponsoring body's press office for advice and support, where there are issues of real or perceived independence, SACs should consider access to independent press advice.

My concerns about SACs have been dismissed on the grounds that I don't understand all the intricacies of the relationships between differently constituted committees. But very few people outside government fully understand these opaque differences, and they are meaningless to the public. As a team at the London School of Economics discovered when trying to generate a list for a 2017 study, it is very difficult to find out how many SACs there are and what each does. They estimated that there were around eighty-three in 2015. There is no clear definition as to what constitutes an SAC, and groups of this type operate under a bewildering array of different names, structures, roles and memberships.

Having separate rules for each committee is a recipe for failure, and is one of the reasons that the current guidance allowing them to use their own press officers is rarely followed. Instead, what we need is a broad principle to affirm that there is a public interest in allowing the public as well as policy makers to see this scientific advice. It could be as simple as saying: 'Independent SACs should be free to publish advice and outputs at a time, and in a manner, of their own choosing.'

There are two important points to make here. Firstly, I am not advocating a free-for-all (or as one comms officer put it, 'letting government advisers talk willy-nilly in the media'). These scientists have access to their own senior science press officers and together they should be trusted to act responsibly in relation to media and liaise with government comms teams when needed. Secondly, I am absolutely not talking about the network of government chief scientific advisers, who work inside Whitehall and so fall into a different category as civil servants. I might love the idea of these people taking to the airwaves regularly, but I understand they could not retain government trust if they did. But that simply does not apply to university academics appointed to supposedly independent SACs, which is why I continue to lobby for change there.

***

David Nutt's fall from grace was not the first time we had experienced a clash between politics and science over independent scientific advice on drugs. In 2008, Professor Sir Michael Rawlins, professor of clinical pharmacology at Newcastle University and chair of the ACMD for many years, asked us to run the committee's press briefings. He felt that holding them in a more independent setting would reinforce the independence of the committee, attracting more science and health reporters, rather than the home affairs journalists who attended when they were held at the Home Office. We took the job on with high hopes, only to find that the reality was much less enjoyable. Home Office press officers who had no relationship with us or the science reporters dictated the timing of briefings, who would be on the panel, who was allowed to do interviews afterwards, which journalists would be invited and every other detail. We dug our heels in and fought, and the hour-long briefing that resulted was just about worth the pain. But in the end, we realised that the SMC's own reputation for independence was being compromised by continuing to be involved, and pulled out.

Some of the government's standard rules for press briefings are ludicrous, and inevitably they irritate journalists. Many are held 'off the record', which means journalists are invited to a press briefing which they cannot report. Others are 'on record' but 'off camera'. I once queried this, asking why they were inviting journalists to a press conference if they didn't want cameras. They explained that if there was a cock-up at the briefing it would be caught on camera, and they did not want footage circulating of a minister looking foolish. After pointing out that these were scientists, not ministers, I suggested that such 'cock-ups' could just as easily be circulated in print or audio in the digital age, but it made no difference. Rules is rules. Another stipulation was that scientists could sit on the panel and speak to a room full of journalists on record for an hour, but must not under any circumstances be interviewed when the hour was finished without it being pre-approved by the departmental press office – who would usually choose the one panel member permitted to speak without bothering to consult the journalists. Dr Adam Rutherford, from BBC Radio 4's *Inside Science*, once went ballistic when he tried to grab a scientist from a panel we had just run on animal research for a quick one-to-one, only to be told by a Home Office press officer that this was simply not allowed.

The other thing government press officers routinely do is break their own embargo by 'trailing' a particular story with a Sunday newspaper. This happened several times when we were hosting briefings with scientists advising government, and we would end up facing a room full of furious science journalists who were being asked to stick to an embargo that had already been broken by those who had set it. Strangely, government press officers never seemed to question this approach, despite the fact that it invariably went wrong for them as overexcited Sunday papers made the most of their exclusives. One backfired in a rather satisfying way for me. We were often asked to run the press briefings for Foresight reports, which were then led by the Government Office for Science (GO-Science). We loved Foresight reports because they brought together the combined expertise of hundreds of the UK's best scientists to look to the future. In 2013, we agreed to run the briefing for the report on land use, on the explicit condition that there was to be no trailing with the Sunday papers. Imagine my surprise when I got a call from Robin McKie at the *Observer* to say he had been offered an exclusive by government press officers for the Sunday before our Monday morning briefing. Robin sympathised with my anger, but wasn't prepared to sacrifice his exclusive. In our ensuing conversation, I just happened to let slip that government comms officers had told me that they didn't want coverage to focus on GM crops. Between us, we decided that it would be most sensible for the *Observer* to focus exclusively on that topic, especially as the daily papers would be directed away from it. The press officers involved were not happy.

There are many and varied examples of how government comms people have managed to thwart the open communication of scientific advice. Another Foresight report, this time on mental health, was delayed repeatedly because special advisers to the prime minister feared that journalists would notice the chapter detailing the evidence of a link between austerity and poor mental health. A report on animal research was delayed because they didn't want it to clash with the prime minister's announcement of a funding boost for Alzheimer's research (I pointed out that most Alzheimer's research uses animals, to no avail). An SMC briefing about Professor Sir Cyril Chantler's report on the effect of plain packaging on the sales of cigarettes was rescheduled to run days earlier than planned, and in Westminster rather than our offices, because the Department of Health needed some distracting news stories that week, while the comms team from the Department for Environment, Food & Rural Affairs (Defra) told Professor Chris Elliott that his independent review of the horsemeat scandal of 2013 was not appropriate for a press briefing, despite a lot of media interest. They also suggested a list of journalists he might like to avoid taking calls from on the launch day – a suggestion he chose to ignore.

These examples may not seem particularly egregious, and I have never argued that government suppresses or manipulates independent scientific advice or the content of these reports. But this is not independent communication of evidence at its best – it's a deliberate politicisation. It chips away at the separation of science and government, and it puts researchers in a difficult position, keen to communicate findings to the public but often not able to challenge government officials. I will continue to lobby for the separation of science from government communications. But it's a battle I have never made any progress on. I felt this particularly keenly during Covid, where all too often the communication of scientific data generated by university academics was 'managed' by government comms officers who tried hard to ensure that the science was aligned with political 'messaging'. But more on that later (see Chapter 11).

Nor have I ever been convinced that this level of control freakery actually benefits the government. Bringing in independent scientists to feed into policy on complex and contentious issues is a good thing for politicians to be doing. So why not be seen to do it? In my endless arguments with government comms people about this, I cite the annual Ipsos MORI Veracity Index surveys, which continue to show that scientists enjoy huge public trust, routinely polling over 80 per cent, while government languishes at the bottom of the table, consistently polling under 25 per cent. I remain convinced that everyone would benefit if we could disrupt the current system to do this differently. Sadly, I have yet to find anyone willing to take on this mammoth task. When former Downing Street chief of staff Dominic Cummings gave his explosive evidence to the joint Covid inquiry of the Health and Social Care and Science and Technology select committees in May 2021, he talked about a deeply ingrained antipathy to openness inside government, and argued that everything about Covid would have been better if the workings of the Scientific Advisory Group for Emergencies (SAGE) and the data it was looking at had been open to scrutiny.

Over the past decade or so, we have occasionally prevailed in our attempts to challenge the status quo – usually when the heads of independent scientific committees were prepared to take a stand. In 2015, Sir Paul Nurse asked us to run the press briefing for his review of the UK's research councils, which he had conducted at the request of the Department for Business, Energy & Industrial Strategy (BEIS). I copied Paul into my many emails refusing to budge on the litany of silly demands coming from the BEIS comms team. He would reply to say simply, 'As Fiona says', and the demands would just fade away. But such victories have been relatively few and far between.

There was one rare and isolated example of an independent SAC that completely bucked the trend. When the SMC opened in 2002, the Royal Commission on Environmental Pollution was one of the most influential and outspoken scientific advisory bodies under its chairman, Professor Sir Tom Blundell. In 2006, his successor Professor Sir John Lawton invited me to address the committee over dinner at The Farmers Club in Whitehall, where its members explained that they had never allowed Defra to launch their reports. After interrogating me to check that the SMC was independent enough to run their briefings, we got the gig. I have used them ever since as proof that the sky doesn't fall in when independent SACs communicate their advice to the media independently from the relevant government department. Sadly, in 2011 the committee became one of the most high-profile victims of the so-called 'Bonfire of the Quangos'. Charles Clover, veteran environment reporter, paid homage to their independent thinking in the *Sunday Times*, though he also suggested that it was the reason they were closed down, which frankly was rather less helpful for my lobbying campaign.

Several years on from the David Nutt affair and the code of practice changes to committees made in its wake, little has changed. That's partly because the scientists who agree to sit on these committees care primarily about whether their advice and recommendations are adopted by governments and serve to inform government policy. They are far less interested in how those findings get into the public domain. Some see their primary function as advising government departments rather than the public, so are prepared to accept the loss of freedom to do media work. Even those who do share my views on this don't want to risk clashing with influential comms advisers attached to the department that they hope will adopt their recommendations.

In September 2014, demoralised by my abject failure to make any progress, I wrote a blog called 'A battle too far?' asking the scientific community if I should give up. The answer in my inbox was loud and crystal clear. We should keep fighting. I printed off the reams of emails, anonymised them and requested a meeting with Dr Claire Craig, a senior policy adviser then working as the director of GO-Science. I headed over to the soulless government building on Victoria Street with a bulging brown envelope of evidence in favour of change. I had put aside an hour for our conversation. It was over within fifteen minutes, before we had even managed to turn on the meeting room lights. She told me that if they had to choose between scientific advice being heard and taken seriously by government versus scientific advice being clearly communicated to the general public via the media, she would always choose the former. I asked why we could not have both; she said that was just the way it was. When I described the meeting to a friend in GO-Science, he said knowingly: 'Ah – a No Coffee meeting.'

***

A separate group of scientists who are also constrained from talking to the media as much as I would like them to are those who work in government-owned laboratories or in arm's-length bodies. They are employed directly by the government and so are technically civil servants. There are thousands of them working in government-owned research institutes, such as Public Health

England's Centre for Radiation, Chemical and Environmental Hazards (CRCE), Defra's Animal and Plant Health Agency (APHA), and the Department of Health's National Institute for Biological Standards and Controls. Most of us have never heard of them, have no idea what they do, nor understand how their work might affect our lives. Sure, their work is published and therefore technically available for perusal, but the reality is most of us can't access or interpret specialist research and journalists simply don't have the time or capacity to read, check and interpret everything – particularly if it's not being proactively distributed. I once posed a Friday afternoon quiz question to science journalists, giving them a long list of these government science agencies and asking which of them they had heard of. It revealed what I had suspected – that many were unaware of the existence of national scientific institutions conducting critical research on many of the most con-tested topics of our times, from vaccine safety to e-cigarettes to animal health.

It would be wrong to say that scientists from these kinds of organisation never speak to the media. A small group of them do, but always in extremely tightly controlled conditions. Government scientists appointed as spokespeople by their institution's comms teams will do lots of media work, especially during a crisis. But they are not free to speak in a way that most people would rec-ognise as open. Journalists cannot simply call them and ask them questions. We cannot add them to our database. If a govern-ment scientist somehow finds their way on to one of our briefing panels, we are quickly reprimanded by senior comms officers for not going through official channels. And when we do go through official channels, we have very little luck: multiple requests over many years to the Public Health England (PHE) comms team for speakers on Novichok, Lyme disease, Zika virus, vaccines, nutri-tion and more have routinely been turned down.

When spokespeople from these agencies do media work, it must go through the central comms team, which is always closely linked to the associated government department comms team. 'Lines' and key messages are agreed before interviews. And government departments decide which agencies take the lead on a particular subject, irrespective of the expertise in those agencies. We were once told during terrible floods that we should stop asking the Met Office for their flooding experts because: 'When water falls as rain, it's a Met Office lead; but when it hits the ground, it's an Environment Agency lead.'

My furious lobbying to liberate these scientists from the clutches of government communications has been one of the most frustrating aspects of my time at the SMC. At one stage in 2018, we were struggling to find toxicologists for our database. The people we had recruited in our early days were gradually moving on to more emeritus positions (an honorary title awarded to retired academics) and therefore distant from the latest research.

I eventually found out via the British Toxicology Society that, for various reasons, much of the toxicology research performed in the UK is done in government labs, especially the CRCE, one of PHE's environmental research sites. One of the society's members was a senior manager from the CRCE, and he invited me to speak to the scientists there, suggesting it would be a great way to recruit new toxicologists to our database. The date was set and I prepared my lecture, packed full of case studies showing that toxicologists engaging with the media could change what the public see and hear for the better. Two days before I was due to speak, the comms team at PHE found out about it. I was asked to submit my slides for vetting. I explained I was happy to show them, but would not be making any changes. Shortly afterwards, the organiser told me that the format for the event had changed: now the CRCE's own comms officer would speak directly after me. That was fine by me; I was delighted they had one and was looking forward to meeting him.

When I arrived, I was staggered by the number of attendees in the lecture theatre. It looked like there were well over two hundred scientists present and I was told the talk was also being live-streamed to others around the country. I felt like a child in a sweet shop. Despite my usual public-speaking nerves, I got off to a flying start, but was rather unnerved by loud sighs coming from the internal comms manager, who was sitting close by me on the stage. The gist of my talk and the examples I showed were to demonstrate that media coverage is more measured and accurate when knowledgeable scientists engage with news reporters. After I sat down, the sighing man jumped to his feet to deliver the exact opposite message, complete with terrifying examples of where government scientists had got things wrong or been double-crossed by journalists. He concluded that only PHE comms people could manage these exchanges, and that all PHE scientists must go through him and the central comms team.

To this day, senior comms managers at PHE and other government agencies assure me that government scientists don't want to speak to the media, and that they are mostly protecting them. I'm sure that's true of many, but it's not true of all. Plus, why would any scientist choose to engage with the media if they knew their press officers felt it was a risky activity that was likely to backfire? Not exactly the moral support and encouragement you would hope to get from your science press office. When I did a similar talk at the Food and Environment Research Agency, a research institute then wholly owned by Defra, several of the scientists I spoke to told me that their induction with the comms team involved a warning never to say anything in public that would embarrass any environment minister. Yet these are scientists, not politicians; and this is the UK, not China.

Interestingly, restrictions on government scientists became a global news story for a while in 2007 when Canada's Prime Minister Stephen Harper introduced new rules preventing federal scientists from speaking to the media without clearance. The move sparked international censure, with editorials in science magazines such as *Nature* condemning the rules, and Canadian scientists fought back and held protests, including a mock funeral for the death of evidence. The restrictions were eventually lifted by Prime Minister Justin Trudeau, shortly after he had won the election in 2015. But throughout all the global outrage on the matter, no one pointed out that the regulations had been identical to the ones we have in the UK.

Another relevant aspect of the thorny issue of governments restricting publicly funded science is the rise of the SPAD inside government. The widespread proliferation of political special advisers brought into government by the party in power is generally traced back to the years of New Labour under Blair and Brown. These politicians had spent so long in the political wilderness that they did not trust the permanent civil servants in the government communications system who had served the Tories for eighteen years, and instead brought in their own advisers including Alastair Campbell and Charlie Whelan. SPADs differ from impartial civil servants in that they are political appointees. David Cameron famously brought in Andy Coulson and Boris Johnson brought in Dominic Cummings. But beneath these well-known names are media SPADs in every department, operating in uneasy alliance with the permanent civil service comms officers. This system matters because these political appointees exert an ever greater influence on government and that trickles down into independent science communication.

One revealing story I heard during Covid was that a leading scientist brought in to help government was told by the BEIS press office that she could not do media interviews about a paper she had written that was being published in the *Lancet*. When she challenged the diktat, she was sent to Lee Cain, Boris Johnson's director of communications and a SPAD himself. Confirming that it was his decision, Cain explained that she was now doing more interviews than most ministers. When I pointed out that Cain was a political SPAD rather than a government comms expert, she looked bewildered. All she knew was that the final decision rested with him, and she did not do the interviews. Another story I heard from a former PHE comms expert was that during the pandemic, when it came to newly published scientific data, instead of coordinating communication and strategy between different departments, it became increasingly common to just receive orders from Number 10 media SPADS without any debate or explanation. That science should be caught up in the government communications system is worrying enough; that decisions about how science is conveyed to the public are now being heavily determined by people who are officially exempt from the civil service's obligations of political impartiality is more so.

It's a continuing source of frustration that I have not been able to get journalists to fully share my concern about this situation. Whenever I discuss it with them, they are briefly outraged. Sometimes they consider how they might report on it. But it generally fits into the 'No shit, Sherlock' category – government press officers are control freaks. It's understandable of course: these journalists typically have to write between three and five stories a day, every day, and can generally find a scientist via us or another press office. They don't have the time to join us in these long-running, time-consuming battles – but I wish they would.

One exception has been the BBC's Pallab Ghosh, who has made it his business to agitate for better access to government scientists. Like many BBC reporters, Ghosh covers a wide brief, but he has long been interested in stories where science meets policy. It was in reaction to news of the devastating fungus known as ash dieback that he and I found ourselves doing battle together side by side.

At that time, a veteran science press officer called Dianne Stilwell had become comms manager at Forest Research, an agency overseen by Defra. It remains unusual for such agencies to recruit people with a science PR background, and she and I were excited by the prospect of working together to get some of these great forest researchers into the media. Soon afterwards, ash dieback hit the UK, and we worked with Stilwell to get a Forest Research expert on the panel of our emergency background briefing on the topic. To our amazement, Stilwell succeeded in persuading Defra to let us have Dr Joan Webber, principal pathologist at Forest Research. One of the UK's most seasoned and experienced tree disease experts, Webber was brilliant on the panel and agreed to be whisked off to the BBC studios at Broadcasting House afterwards with Ghosh and his producer to do another set of interviews. Then the fun started.

We were contacted by press officers at Defra furious that we had put their expert into the hands of the BBC. We explained that she had received permission from their press office to take part; they replied that this extended only to the briefing, not to interviews afterwards. At Broadcasting House, Ghosh and his producer were having lunch with Webber in between interviews when she showed them both a text from a Defra comms officer instructing her to cancel any planned interviews and leave the building. Shortly afterwards, Defra staff arrived at the BBC in person, took Webber to one side and again advised that she not do any further interviews. When she and I spoke about it at length a month or so later, Webber told me how the incident was the culmination of a long period of increasing restrictions on scientists from

Forest Research speaking to journalists. In her early years there, she often answered the phone to reporters and enjoyed talking to them. Then a new rule was introduced requiring scientists to seek prior permission before any interactions with journalists. Whenever she asked, she was either denied permission or it came too late to be of use. Not surprisingly journalists eventually stopped calling her. There was no gagging order, but Defra's activities had had the same effect.

The increasing problem of centralised control was later acknowledged publicly by Lord Smith, who chaired the Environment Agency after leaving the Commons. Writing in 2017, after he had stepped down as chair, Smith said that the agency's core role was to be an independent, impartial adviser to government but that this function had been curtailed by politicians under Cameron's coalition government:

> It was made very clear to us that, whilst private impartial advice was still sought and still welcome, it should not under any circumstances be put into the public domain. It was up to ministers to decide what the public should be told, not up to us. And we did what we were told; we had no other option.

He went on to reiterate the vital need for 'the painstaking assembly of, and restatement of, evidence, fact and truth' in a world where people seemed increasingly keen to dismiss evidence and expertise.

The number of people willing to criticise this trend publicly is tiny, however. After what happened to Joan Webber on the ash dieback story, Ghosh set out to write a feature on the problem. I gave him plenty of names of scientists and science press officers I knew had had similar experiences, but none of them agreed to go on the record. In the end, I was the only person prepared to do so.

He had to embroider my status considerably to get the piece published. Under the headline 'Call to let government scientists off the leash' Ghosh's top line read: 'One of the UK's most influential science communicators is pressing the government to let more of its scientists speak to the media.' Despite my lifelong aversion to hype, I rather enjoyed my elevation.

My reputation for lobbying on this issue led to an invitation from Professor Bill Sutherland, then the president of the British Ecology Society, to deliver a keynote speech at its annual conference. I deliberately didn't use the word 'gagged' in my talk because I don't think it's the right word. There is no official gagging order and, as I've said, some government scientists do lots of media work under controlled conditions. But the term came up in a comment from the floor, and after my speech I was surrounded by scientists from a variety of government agencies. It was like being at an AA meeting as they introduced themselves to me: 'My name is Giles, and I am gagged.' Buoyed by the event, one of the affected scientists invited me to her agency to do a talk. I called her several days later to arrange a date. She sounded nervous and asked if she could call back later. Ringing from outside her office, she said that she had raised the idea with the comms team, and it had not gone down well . . .

I occasionally ask the SMC's board of trustees and advisers if we should give up trying to change this situation. It felt like an entirely fruitless and frustrating endeavour, and it had been made clear to me that certain important supporters of science within government didn't appreciate our efforts. If we were making any kind of difference, I would have put up with upsetting people; but if anything the problem appears to be growing. Adopting a rather pessimistic attitude, my board generally urges us to keep up the pressure, on the basis that we might at least stop things getting even worse.

In March 2015, Cabinet Secretary Sir Jeremy Heywood sent a letter to research councils and other scientific institutions around the UK to alert them to a proposed amendment to the Civil Service Code that would require all civil servants to seek ministerial authorisation before 'any contact with the media in an official capacity'. A year later, the government announced the anti-lobbying clause, designed to stop organisations in receipt of government grants from lobbying government for change. The changes would have applied to publicly funded scientists working for government labs and any university academics who receive government funding for their work. Many comms managers simply sent emails alerting scientists to the coming changes. Others, however, shared our concern. Sense About Science, Stempra (the science comms PR network) and the Campaign for Science and Engineering joined us in kicking up a major stink, organising joint letters and lobbying scientists in government to resist the changes. Thankfully both proposals eventually died a death, but the fact that senior people in government and the civil service thought these were a good idea – on top of all the restrictions and controls already in place – showed that constant vigilance was necessary.

One of my few personal triumphs in this arena has been getting 'purdah' rules changed. The term is used by government to refer to a pre-election period of reduced communication from government that applies to civil servants working inside government and in 'arm's length bodies' (ALBs). It is intended to avoid conferring political advantage on any one party, and should simply mean that major funding announcements or corporate campaigns are postponed until after an election. So far, so sensible. But in the early 2010s, we noticed more and more scientists citing purdah as a reason to avoid speaking to journalists. Scientists in research council units and laboratories such as the MRC's Laboratory of Molecular Biology or the Natural Environment Research

Council's British Antarctic Survey told us that, a decade ago, they were encouraged to carry on as normal during elections. Now, however, they were on the receiving end of ever more cautious guidance sent by comms staff in government departments and their own research councils.

At its worst, the overreach of purdah into day-to-day science has seen independent scientists not publicising their own findings and refusing to comment on breaking news. In 2017 I organised a joint letter to the Cabinet Office, signed by representatives from fourteen scientific bodies, protesting the mission creep of purdah. After years of being ignored on this subject by government and media alike, I remember the sheer joy of reading the leader in *The Times* that followed. Under the title 'Gagged Science', the editorial alluded to the madness of the Met Office refusing to comment on a global warming story for fear of being seen as political, and said:

> As taxpayers, Britons spend billions on government-sponsored scientific research and expertise. As voters, we are denied the benefit of that expertise by rules intended to keep civil servants out of politics at election time. This makes no sense. Scientists, with few exceptions, are not civil servants . . . Scientists do not belong in purdah.

Sue Gray was once described by a journalist as 'the most powerful person you have never heard of in government'. People laugh when I describe her as the 'Head of Purdah', but as director general of the propriety and ethics team at the Cabinet Office, she was indeed the person in charge of it. With the help of the Institute for Government and the Royal Statistical Society, which were both concerned about this issue, I met her to discuss it. Gray made two things completely clear to me: that she was a passionate believer in purdah; but also that it was never intended to apply to independent scientists doing business as usual. She and I had several exchanges about how best to enshrine the principles of academic freedom within purdah rules. In early 2018, Gray called me as I was walking on a beach in Ireland to report that she had just finalised the official guidance and had made two changes that she hoped would stop purdah encroaching on the freedom of speech of university scientists. It was music to my ears: a clause stating clearly and categorically that purdah rules do not apply to independent academics going about their daily work:

> The principles set out here are not about restricting commentary from independent sources, for example academics who may also hold public appointments or non-executive roles in government departments or public bodies. It is for individual public bodies to apply this pre-election guidance within their own organisations, but in doing so, they should not go beyond the principles set out in this document.

I was ecstatic. I called the office and asked them to put me on speaker phone. 'I think we may have fixed purdah!' I shouted down the phone, to screams of delight from my colleagues.

In all my time campaigning against purdah overreach, I never met anyone who thought it was a good thing. But it tells you a lot about how the system works that something that no one agrees with can become the norm. The problem was that it was no one's job to stop it. This was a small but significant victory in the broader battle.

As I write, there are other glimmers of hope. In 2019, Professor Gideon Henderson was appointed as Defra's new chief scientific adviser. I asked for an early meeting, and bent his ear about the silencing of scientists working at Defra research institutes. Just weeks after our meeting, Professor Henderson saw what I was talking about first-hand when Defra's press team tried to pull a scientist from the Animal and Plant Health Agency (APHA) off the panel for a press briefing on new research on badgers and TB. Over a weekend off, he intervened and the briefing went ahead with the panel unchanged. Following that incident, he invited me to a meeting with some senior comms officers in Defra, where I suggested a pilot scheme to allow a small number of APHA scientists onto our database to be treated in the same way as their academic counterparts. The simple test: would the sky fall in if these scientists engaged with the media? Eighteen months after this suggestion was first made, we learned in May 2021 that the pilot could go ahead. Several months after the emergence of Covid, PHE press officers approached us to ask if we would host some media briefings for their scientists. Is the Pope a Catholic? For a decade, we had been trying to get senior government scientists on to SMC briefings. I wish it had not taken a national pandemic, in which all the old rules were torn up, to get it.

I may not sound like a huge fan of government press officers, but I don't blame them for the situation I have described here. Many are smart and have great integrity. Nor do I doubt that government press officers do a good job for ministers. It's the way that impartial and objective scientific evidence and expertise get caught up in a system designed for politics that causes me concern. Under the 'What we do' section of the Government Communication Service website, the remit of government communicators is spelled out: 'Our goal is to provide an exceptional standard of professional practice to support the government, implementing the priorities of the Prime Minister and the Cabinet to build a stronger economy, a fairer society, a United Kingdom and a global Britain.'

In September 2021, the Institute for Government (IfG) published a guest paper by Lee Cain, who had left the government by then, that argued that unclear lines of responsibility and mixed messages from different government departments undermined the government's Covid response. Cain's insight into the thinking at the highest level of government communications confirmed my worst fears. His argument was that government would have done a better job on the pandemic if everyone linked with government was speaking with 'one voice' under central direction. But many of those linked with government during Covid were research scientists working for publicly funded bodies such as UK Research and Innovation and PHE, or university academics. Far from seeing them as apolitical actors, Cain argued that independent communications from these ALBs had been problematic:

> All too often during the pandemic, government communication plans were knocked off course by briefings from within ALBs that had not been shared with central government ... This could have been solved by having a closer relationship, and a clearer command and control structure, between government and ALBs, with clearer understanding of clearance processes.

I was really pleased that the IfG published Cain's paper to open up public debate, because these discussions matter to us all. I draw the opposite conclusions from him. Mixed messages and public confusion can be harmful, but the Covid pandemic has demonstrated that the public can be trusted to absorb uncertainty and make judgements in the face of complexity. Explaining preliminary and contradictory science is messy; that should not be seen as a failure of communications.

People who have become weary of my lobbying on this ask

me to prove why the current system is so wrong. I have plenty of examples of how I think it could be improved to better serve the public interest, but I want to ask them a question in return. What is so wrong with allowing independent scientists who volunteer to advise government or gather data at the request of government to communicate that science themselves? I have yet to hear a convincing answer.

In the end, I think any major change to the culture within government communications will have to come from senior politicians or the civil service. I once asked Sue Gray what the sanction against scientists who broke purdah was – were they sent to the Tower of London? She laughed and said she wasn't aware there had ever been sanctions. Maybe, in the end, scientists all need to follow Sir Paul Nurse's example, and just say no. The loss of control might be painful for a while, but I bet government would reap the benefits many times over in terms of public trust.

6

SCIENTISTS V SCEPTICS

The story of Climategate

EVERY SO OFTEN, a story comes along that is so messy, politicised and toxic that all the principles of open engagement go out the window. One of these stories was the affair in 2009 that became known as 'Climategate' – when unknown hackers dumped ten years' worth of email exchanges between leading climate scientists on to the internet. Researchers recoiled in horror as sceptics highlighted the messages that painted climate science in the worst possible light and managed to garner enormous coverage in the world's media. Many feared that the controversy would prove the death knell for public trust in climate science and a major setback for those relying on the credibility of the science to convince policymakers that action was needed to reduce CO_2 emissions.

I don't actually remember how I found out about the hacked emails, although they dominated life at the SMC for many months; it's one of the stories that left its mark on everyone who got involved. That was nothing, however, compared to its effect on the scientist at the centre of the storm. In November 2009, Professor Phil Jones, director of the Climatic Research Unit (CRU) at the University of East Anglia (UEA), learned – along with the rest of the world – that a large number of his emails and documents, covering over thirteen years of research, had been stolen. The emails were leaked to a website just days before a major climate summit in Copenhagen. Climate change sceptics were quick to seize on them and, within days, their interpretation of the emails moved from the blogosphere to become the dominant narrative in the global media: that they revealed a vast conspiracy to over-state the scientific case for global warming and suppress contrary findings. These emails proved what they had been saying all along, they argued – that climate change was a hoax.

We swung into action. Our first thought was to get Jones on a train and into the SMC. Whatever the truth, we knew we needed him to interpret his own emails rather than leave it to his critics. Our phones were on fire with science reporters desperate to hear from him, so I called Simon Dunford, our main contact in the UEA press team. Dunford and his boss Annie Ogden seemed to share our view that we needed to get Jones out there to explain his own emails. But they could not deliver. The university was officially treating the hack as a crime and was asking the media and others not to report on the emails because they were stolen property. The police were investigating and there would be no comment from Professor Jones or anyone else. So, no, they could not get him on a train to us.

We were dismayed. We understood how difficult it was, but every screen in our office had the talking head of a familiar climate sceptic gleefully quoting decontextualised extracts. Their favourite email was from Jones to US climatologist Professor Michael Mann in 1999, in which he discussed what he called Mann's '*Nature* trick' to 'hide the decline' in global warming – seemingly a smoking gun for anyone who didn't believe in climate change. Jones's colleagues, however, told us that the 'trick' simply involved using data from a longer period of time to properly demonstrate the historic heat rise. Other exchanges were selected to show how Jones and his colleagues were working out ways to keep inconvenient findings out of peer-reviewed journals, and were downplaying scientific disagreements about Mann's famous 'hockey stick' graph, which had been widely cited as demonstrating that global warming in the twentieth century had been unprecedented. Used out of context, Jones's words were alleged to prove that he and other researchers were fiddling data and the press was having a field day. 'The big climate change fraud' was the front page of the *Daily Express*.

The press officers at UEA sounded as dismayed as us that they could not get Phil Jones into the SMC to answer for his own emails. So much of the UK's world-class climate research took place at UEA that the press team there were specialists in climate science comms. I got the distinct impression that the media strategy for this crisis was being dictated by people way above the paygrade of the media team. In my experience, that is never a good thing. The further up the communications ladder you go in universities, the further you move away from the science press officers who understand the material they're dealing with. The directors of corporate communications, and the crisis management agencies they often employ at times like this, are tasked with protecting the reputation of the institution; the public's understanding of science is not their primary concern. But this was building up to be a global media storm, which threatened to derail the Copenhagen climate summit and undermine public trust in the scientific consensus on climate change, as well as trust in science more generally. There was a much bigger issue at stake than the reputation of a single university.

Professor Jones's research area involves measuring the annual growth rings in ancient trees to assess historic temperature change. As this relatively esoteric background might suggest, he is a mild-mannered man who does not enjoy the media limelight, and he was certainly not mentally prepared to be in it for all the wrong reasons. The media circus around Jones grew rapidly, with journalists camped outside his house and doorstepping his neighbours; he received hundreds of abusive emails; and threats were made against him and his family. We had no idea at the time just how great a toll the scandal was having on him. A decade later, when a prime-time BBC drama told the story of Climategate, a former colleague of Jones told me that the speed at which he had collapsed was astonishing: he lost a lot of weight very rapidly and was hardly able to talk – he became almost 'ghost-like'.

I suspect the UEA leadership team probably did not know what to make of the emails in those critical early days. In many ways, it was to UEA's great credit that the institution refused to rush to judgement, wanting instead to give its employee due process and consistently prioritising its duty of care for him. But sitting in the SMC in London, UEA's response felt slow and inadequate. The idea that journalists would postpone their reporting until the crime was solved, or UEA's investigation concluded, was completely naive. I felt then – and now – that the best thing those senior academics could have done was to listen to their media team.

In the absence of a response from Jones, we entreated climate scientists to send us comments or speak to journalists, regardless of their views on the controversy. We explained that they didn't have to address the detailed content of the emails or defend Professor Jones. We simply needed them to emphasise what was already known about climate science and to explain that, even if it were true that Jones's datasets had been manipulated, there were plenty of other reliable datasets showing the same impacts. Some brave scientists agreed, and on the day the story broke, we sent eight comments out to journalists. Some simply stressed the overwhelming scale and consistency of the evidence of climate change available from a wide variety of sources. Others directly addressed the emails, but dismissed the idea that they proved anything about the state of the science. Some went further, defending what they had seen of the leaked correspondence as part and parcel of a robust scientific debate. Professor John Burrows, from the Centre for Ecology & Hydrology, said:

> The peer review scientific process was created to try to avoid conspiracies from any side on an issue. Despite the adverse reaction in some quarters, the current discussion is a good example that, whilst it doesn't always look perfect, an open debate, backed up by peer review, is what science is all about.

One of the comments we offered came from a non-scientist, Bob Ward, who was by then head of policy and comms for the Grantham Research Institute on Climate Change and the Environment, at the London School of Economics and Political Science (LSE). One of the SMC's policies is that we usually only ask scientists expert in the correct field to comment on an issue, but we felt this particular crisis was an exception. There were elements of this story that were not only about the science, but also the conduct of climate scientists and science communication. By this point, Ward was already one of the more influential and visible climate communicators in the UK, appearing regularly in print since 2005, when in his former role as comms director for the Royal Society he called for ExxonMobil to stop misrepresenting climate science. He was also something that most senior climate scientists were not – available and willing.

In the hours and days after the story broke, Ward almost single-handedly filled the vacuum left in the UK's TV and radio studios by the majority of the UK's climate scientists and official climate research agencies. All day long, the screens in our office showed him going from Sky, to the BBC, to ITN, defending climate science and doing battle with the sceptics. I don't always agree with Ward, and a few eminent climate scientists have queried his credentials as an expert speaker on climate science. But he took to the studios back then because not enough climate scientists were willing to do so, and because he feared climate science would pay a high price for leaving an empty chair. I always felt Ward was driven by that fear rather than his ego – a suspicion strengthened a few years later when we invited him to speak at an event for scientists new to media work. Ward showed the 200-strong audience a clip of an interview he had given during that period, where he visibly lost his temper in a discussion with Fraser Nelson, the editor of the *Spectator*. His self-deprecating advice for the audience? 'Never lose your temper live on air – it's not a good look.'

The hacking of Jones's email account came at a time of open warfare between the climate science community and climate sceptics – a period covered in Fred Pearce's excellent book *The Climate Files*, which shows how years of obsessive or malicious Freedom of Information (FOI) requests from climate change deniers had taken its toll on researchers like Jones. As Pearce puts it:

> The clash between the blogosphere and the pages of august journals such as *Nature* could not be greater. But within it is a Shakespearean tragedy of misunderstood motives. The bunker mentality – of climate scientists faced with the mob trying to take over their labs – is brutally exposed in the emails. But so too is the opportunism of the outsiders and the confusion caused in the labs by their efforts to question what was going on.

There were moments of light relief or, I suppose, occasional missteps, depending on your perspective. Professor Andy Watson was one of the few UEA scientists who agreed to do media interviews. He had read the hacked emails and was prepared to address them directly. In a testy exchange with leading American sceptic Marc Morano on *Newsnight*, Watson made his point succinctly: 'Despite the best efforts of the sceptics, there is no instance in these emails that anyone has found so far – and there are millions of people looking – that suggests the scientists manipulated their fundamental data.' As the interview finished, I was midway through a text to congratulate him when, with cameras still rolling, Watson said audibly on air of his opponent: 'What an arsehole.'

The weeks after the release of the emails were a challenging time at the SMC. We turned our attention towards the climate science big hitters. We approached the chief scientists and heads of the Met Office, the Natural Environment Research Council (NERC), and the Grantham Institutes at both LSE and Imperial College London. Again, our pitch was that they did not need to explain Jones's emails or defend him, but they were desperately needed to defend the overall quality of climate research and state clearly which evidence could be relied on, which bits were more uncertain and which questions were yet to be answered. We were trying to persuade them that engaging and embracing this controversy was the 'God-given' opportunity to get their science across that Tim Radford had described years earlier to GM researchers. But few had the appetite to embrace this controversy. Others simply didn't see it as their responsibility. I remember calling the head of press at a university that boasted lots of climate scientists to ask what she could do. She replied that there were also climate sceptics among their academics, so she didn't feel this was something with which she should get involved.

I hoped to get a better response from NERC – after all, this was the body responsible for the grants of public money that funded a huge portion of the UK's climate science. We thought that the attack on the integrity of that science should have been keeping their head of communications awake at night. It was – but not in quite the way I was hoping for. When I called to find out what they were thinking about media, she told me that things had got so bad that she had stopped telling people where she worked. A very senior member of UEA later told me that, when the university asked government, NERC and the Met Office for support, they were told that these three powerful bodies had all decided to 'hunker down' and let UEA deal with the crisis. It was this kind of response that led Bob Ward to describe Climategate as 'a shameful episode for the climate research community, which largely hid from view. It was a disgraceful display of spinelessness and incompetence.'

UEA did start to put up senior representatives to do media work, including their vice-chancellor Professor Edward Acton and leading scientists such as Professor Bob Watson, a former climate adviser to the US government. They also finally put Jones up to do a single interview about a week after the leak was revealed, with Emily Beament, the environment correspondent at the Press Association. The professor stood by the science conducted at his unit, categorically denying the claims that climate data was being manipulated. But he also expressed regret at some of the emails he had sent, admitting to using 'poorly chosen words in the heat of the moment, when I was frustrated'. Re-reading that interview now I am struck by how robust he was in defending both his science and his integrity. This was no mealy-mouthed attempt to explain away the indefensible. Yet in the febrile atmosphere of the time, doing just one interview felt like a spectacularly inadequate response to the global fire storm.

In January 2010, another scandal hit climate science when it was discovered that a claim in the 2007 report from the Intergovernmental Panel on Climate Change (IPCC) was inaccurate. The claim – that Himalayan glaciers could be near to disappearing by 2035 – was traced by *New Scientist* to an interview it had conducted with an Indian glaciologist in 1999. But it was not backed up in any peer-reviewed study, and was rebuffed by other glaciologists, who maintained that the glaciers could take centuries to vanish. This time, there were calls for the head of the IPCC, Dr Rajendra Pachauri, to resign. Kelvin MacKenzie, former editor of the *Sun*, wrote: 'I'm delighted to report that going up in smoke on the global warming bonfire are the careers of lying professors, deceitful glaciologists, rainforest racketeers, and our old friends the bandwagon politicians.'

If there was anything good to come of what inevitably became known as 'Glaciergate', it was that our ever more desperate pleas to the big hitters finally began to be heard. We set up a briefing for early February with three eminent and influential climate scientists: Professor Dame Julia Slingo, chief scientist at the Met Office; Professor Alan Thorpe, chief executive of NERC; and Professor Sir Brian Hoskins, director of the Grantham Institute for Climate Change at Imperial. By that point, several science journalists had confided that they were being accused by their editors of having 'gone native', with the implication that they had become so close to the researchers they were no longer able to scrutinise the science objectively. These science reporters arrived at the SMC in a slightly agitated state, feeling as though their necks were on the chopping block if they didn't go back to their offices with a powerful response from the science establishment. One told me that when he told his editor he hadn't been aware that IPCC reports sometimes included 'grey literature' (non-peer-reviewed material, which is therefore considered less authoritative than research subject to the peer review process), the response was: 'Well, we fucking employ you to know that stuff.' It all made for an interesting atmosphere at the briefing

– the first time members of the UK climate science community had made themselves so available to science journalists since the hack in November.

There were nineteen agitated science and environment journalists in the room that morning, from all of the UK's main news outlets. Steve Connor, science editor of the *Independent*, summed up the mood in the room when he saw me heading over to have a quick behind-the-scenes chat with the scientists and heckled me: 'Fiona – this better be good!' Imagine my dismay, then, when I walked into the green room to have the scientists tell me they would not under any circumstances answer any questions about Professor Jones's emails or whether Dr Pachauri should resign from the IPCC. I accepted that they were here to speak about the strength of the global scientific evidence base for climate change; I wanted them to do that. But we had called this press conference in response to the crisis caused by the hacked emails and the row over the IPCC's report. I argued that they would have to acknowledge and address the issues raised in the emails since these would likely make up most of the journalists' questions. I also argued that there were ways of answering these questions that avoided getting into the specifics of some of the more unsavoury messages. But they were adamant, and it was clear that they had already discussed the matter among themselves. In the end, the scientists probably did me a favour. While I felt under pressure from the journalists next door to deliver some kind of 'fight back', I had consistently argued that the challenge for the climate science community was to convey the strength of their findings to the wider public and policy makers. Headlines defending Jones or Pachauri might have been popular with the journalists, but I wanted headlines defending the integrity of climate research. Still, at the time it was with some trepidation I led them into what felt like the lion's den.

Before taking questions the panellists gave a presentation that looked at which parts of climate science were well-established fact, which were more uncertain and open to debate, and which bits remained unknown. They also talked about how the science was conducted, the kinds of peer review process at work, the way research is selected for funding, and the myriad ways in which quality is achieved. They acknowledged that they hadn't always communicated effectively the uncertainties inherent in climate science, leaving the public understandably confused. After a week in which poor-quality science, flaws in peer review and academic errors had loomed large in the media, they argued forcefully that we must not throw the baby out with the bathwater. I loved it.

But it wasn't good enough for the hacks. Many of them wanted robust defences of Jones's emails, and specifics about the offending messages, but the panel refused to be drawn. Michael McCarthy, the *Independent*'s environment editor, took to his feet and, to nods of agreement all round, asked slightly incredulously: 'Is this it? Is this the fightback?' Another reporter said: 'We came here to get the final nail in the climate sceptics' coffin, but all you've done is tell us what the evidence says.' To which the scientists replied: 'Yes – we're scientists. That's what we do.' As the journalists trailed out of the briefing, the consensus was that scientists were going to have to up their game if they were to win back public and media trust.

It was an unusual situation. The journalists were frustrated with the scientists and with us. I should have been dismayed, but actually I was proud. There are always risks to sitting in front of a room full of journalists in the middle of a media frenzy, and the briefing itself was not comfortable. But sometimes, risks are worth taking. Under the headline 'Global warming is full of uncertainties and the public is right to be confused, scientists admitted today', Mike Swain, the *Daily Mirror*'s science reporter, wrote a clear, nuanced account of the briefing, setting out the consensus that existed and explaining why uncertainties remained. He quoted Professor Sir Brian Hoskins as saying, among other points: 'I am sometimes asked if I believe in climate change. It isn't a question of belief. This is science. The pressure all the time is to try to reduce the uncertainty, but it will always remain. Climate is a chaotic system and there will always be uncertainties.' It was perfect. No false equivalence, or sceptics trying to politicise the subject and spread misinformation. No diversions into the offending emails. Just wall-to-wall climate science. And in a mass-readership red top.

Some years later, I was invited to address the NERC board about media work, and I used that climate briefing as a case study on the benefits of embracing controversy. Professor Duncan Wingham, who had replaced Alan Thorpe as chief executive, told those assembled that some of his colleagues had been very unhappy about the briefing, and he felt it would have been better for NERC to stay well out of the fray. Discovering that the current head of NERC took a dim view of one of the few bold media interventions the science community had made, and that presumably he would not have been on the panel had Climategate happened on his watch, was depressing.

Climategate arrived at a time when influential voices, especially campaigners who wanted governments to combat climate change, were reacting badly to any questioning of climate science. Some went as far as suggesting that the evidence for climate change was so well-established that the media shouldn't even be debating it. They argued that scientists should stop talking about the uncertainties because they were being seized on by sceptics as a means of fostering doubt among the wider general public.

I saw two problems here. Firstly, I was wary of the 'good lie', where you downplay differences of opinion or uncertainties for the greater good; it so often backfires, and critics are then able to use this lack of honesty and transparency to discredit research. Secondly, I hate it when scientists do anything based on how their critics will react. (One thing that Professor Jones's emails did show was how a lot of climate scientists had become utterly obsessed with their tormentors, seeing everything through their eyes.) I spend a considerable amount of my life asking scientists to put such thoughts to one side and instead focus on the general public who deserve to hear the truth and who can generally be trusted to cope with the nuances. My argument is that if scientists are not open about uncertainties, differences of opinion, mistakes and findings that challenge the consensus, it will give sceptics the advantage of gleefully 'revealing the truth'. Great science will win out only if the public trusts that the scientists are telling the truth and playing it straight. Many researchers came round to this point of view and we ran press conferences addressing various issues: the alleged 'pause' in global warming; errors in one of the IPCC reports; and the suggestion in a *Nature* geoscience paper that we might have more time than previously thought before we exceed 1.5°C of warming.

At the SMC, we have always tried to be a press office that embraces debate rather than attempting to close it down. Over the years we have defended the rights of the BBC and others to include other voices in debates on climate change. We shared the wider frustration at the 'false balance' that characterised early coverage of climate change, and often argued with journalists that their choice of sceptics to fuel a media 'row' was lazy and unlikely to help their audiences to gain a better understanding of the topic. But claiming that any field of science is 'settled' or beyond debate is fundamentally unscientific. '*Nullius in verba*', the Royal Society's motto, means 'take nobody's word for it', a nod to a proud tradition of scepticism in science. Attempting to close down debate is also just a terrible look. 'The public must believe this because scientists say so' just doesn't feel right in today's less deferential world. In some ways, Climategate was a healthy corrective to a community that had become accustomed to making pronouncements rather than engaging in a wider debate. In an editorial published on 23 November 2009, the *Financial Times* summed up my view perfectly:

> [Scientists] must not react to unpopularity by closing ranks against a hostile world or by feeling obliged to campaign for the cause. Although the dividing line between research and campaigning can be hard to distinguish, scientists must try to respect it. Their value rests above all in the ability to provide evidence as objectively as possible. Politicians, businesses and environmental groups can then pick up the scientific evidence and base policies on it.

Well said. The public had already benefited enormously from scientists engaging in open debate with opponents of GM and human–animal hybrids and, uncomfortable as it was, the time had come for climate scientists to do the same.

Of course, it takes two to tango. If some scientists had been keen to keep the complex uncertainties of climate science behind closed doors, sections of the media were also guilty of glossing over uncertainties in the pursuit of dramatic headlines. In 2006, the respected Institute for Public Policy Research published a report talking about how alarmist language leads to 'climate porn'. I recognised the concept – indeed, we were arguably responsible for creating some of it. I remember a press briefing in January 2005 on a significant new *Nature* paper on levels of warming. The study showed that we could be facing increases in warming of anything between 2°C and 11°C by 2100. In emails and meetings beforehand, I repeatedly warned the authors that the media would all go with the maximum figure as their top line. They responded by explaining that this top line would be entirely misleading and inaccurate because the statistically significant models were mostly clustered around the 2 to 3°C mark. I urged them to emphasise the lower number repeatedly: I knew of no self-respecting sub-editor who would use a more modest number in their headline when a bigger scarier one was on offer. But it didn't make any difference. As I chaired the briefing, I smiled wryly at question after question about whether, if warming increased by 11°C, London would disappear into the oceans or freeze over as it did in the Hollywood movie *The Day After Tomorrow*, which had been released the previous year. The next day, I got on the tube to see London's commuters reading the *Metro* as usual. The front page had a huge 11°C beneath a murky picture of an industrial facility pumping black smoke into a sky, with 'That's how much hotter scientists believe world will get ... and it will be worse in Britain' emblazoned in large text next to the number.

Before Climategate, it often felt as though journalists at our climate briefings would mentally start packing up as soon as they got their 'worse than previously expected' or 'beyond the tipping point' headlines. I remember the first 'normal' climate press briefing after the controversy, in March 2010. It was to promote a new study on the human imprint of climate change, led by Dr Peter Stott from the Met Office. Separating the human contribution to warming from natural variability is complicated science, and this was a significant breakthrough in understanding. But instead of rushing back to file the story, the journalists loitered well beyond the usual hour, pressing the authors on what the science showed and interrogating every data point. This side effect felt positive to us. The best climate scientists had nothing to fear from much more intense scrutiny, and Stott was in his element under heavy questioning. The general public benefited from comprehensive, reliable reporting as opposed to climate porn or a 'he said, she said' story. Win win.

In the years since the Climategate scandal broke, there has been much discussion within mainstream science about whether the media was wrong to give the hacking story such prominence. With hindsight, it's easier to say that this whole saga was a non-story. But even at the time there were several voices making that argument. Dr Myles Allen, a climate scientist from the University of Oxford, and Dr David Adam, the *Guardian*'s environment reporter, argued from day one that the hack had been politically motivated by activists trying to wreck the Copenhagen climate summit. Allen criticised 'the spectacular failure of mainstream journalism to keep the whole affair in perspective'. Others agreed. Former green activist Mark Lynas argued in the *New Statesman* that reporting the emails was giving in to the 'barbarians at the gate'. And Elizabeth May, long-serving leader of the Green Party in Canada, wrote: 'How dare the world's media fall into the trap set by contrarian propagandists.'

I understand where the proponents of this argument are coming from, but my opinion differs. With silence from Professor Jones in the early days, and a huge cache of seemingly incriminating material, it was simply too good a story for any journalist to miss. Secondly, it felt to me like the worst time possible for scientists to suggest that climate science should be somehow immune to investigative journalism. As I wrote at the time, it is precisely because climate change is so important that it requires rigorous, robust investigative journalism. Any reporting that gives climate science an easy ride simply plays into the sceptics' hands. Finally, I still believe the scandal, like all media storms, provided an opportunity to communicate climate science. Fred Pearce's investigative work shone a massive light on climate science and revealed weaknesses, flaws and rivalries. But it also found climate research in rude health. His conclusion: 'Have the Climategate revelations undermined the case that we are experiencing man-made climate change? Absolutely not.' Michael Hanlon, something of a climate sceptic himself in his early days of reporting on the issue, covered the story for the *Daily Mail* and said, after he managed to read all the emails, 'Scratch and sniff as we did, there was no smoking gun, no line that would show that there had been a conspiracy to fabricate a Great Untruth.' From the *Guardian* to the *Daily Mail*, journalists combed through those emails for evidence that climate science was a hoax, but failed to find any. It may have been disproportionate to look that hard, but it may perhaps have resulted in strengthening public trust in climate scientists rather than the reverse.

Several official enquiries went on to clear Professor Phil Jones and the CRU of all the substantive charges. He was criticised for trying to avoid releasing emails under FOI, and for the tone of some of the emails, but none of the independent investigations found anything that indicated scientists had manipulated the evidence on climate change. The SMC ran the press conferences for three of these inquiries, as well as a press conference for UEA's vice-chancellor to respond to its conclusions. The one we were most closely involved in was the review chaired by Sir Muir Russell, commissioned by UEA as a wholly independent inquiry. The PR agency employed by Russell turned out to be Luther Pendragon, run by Mike Granatt, a former head of government communications and one of the SMC's founding board members. Granatt is, in my view, a communications genius, and I was thrilled when he invited the SMC to run the press launch. But he also invited me to meet the inquiry team and watch them at work. This was by far the most rigorous of the inquiries, and I was impressed by both the huge amount of time and dedication the panel members invested in doing their job and the impartiality they demonstrated. However, a question about their impartiality led to one sticky moment.

Dr Philip Campbell, then editor-in-chief of *Nature*, was one of the few scientists appointed to the Russell review. Campbell and I were friends, and I was horrified when he called to tell me that he was about to resign from the review panel. He had visited China soon after the hack and, before he had been invited to join the inquiry team, had given a late-night interview in which he told a Chinese journalist that Jones and the other scientists were 'behaving as researchers should'. That quote had been unearthed by climate sceptics, who claimed he had pre-empted the outcome of the inquiry. On the evening the news broke, I was actually on a bus on my way to Campbell's house to have dinner with him and a few other friends, a journey I spent fending off calls from journalists asking for reaction to news of his resignation. One call came literally as I was ringing his doorbell. It was Jonathan Amos, long-time science correspondent at the BBC, asking if I had any idea where he could find Campbell. I was still on the phone as the man in question opened his door, so I put my finger over my mouth to shush him while apologising to Amos for not being able to help. Later that evening, Campbell and I left his other guests and took our wine to his front room to watch his resignation discussed on *Newsnight*.

I didn't make it through Climategate without my own slip-up. Early in 2010, I had finished a report on the future of science and the media commissioned by the science minister Lord Drayson, and was thrilled when *The Media Show* on BBC Radio 4 asked me in to talk about our findings. When I arrived, I discovered that I was to follow a pre-record with arch-sceptic James Delingpole about the BBC's coverage of climate change. The first question I was asked was how I would have handled the media work around Professor Jones's emails. Caught on the hop, I said I would have done things very differently from the UEA media team and instead persuaded Jones to do a round of interviews explaining his own emails and challenging any misleading interpretations. I drew a contrast between Jones's lack of engagement and Professor David Nutt's response to his sacking, when he had done back-to-back interviews defending his science to great effect. By this point in the scandal, influential environmental columnist for the *Guardian* George Monbiot had publicly called on both Professor Jones and then Annie Ogden, the head of UEA communications, to resign. I disagreed with him on both counts, yet here I was, disparaging UEA's media strategy live on BBC Radio 4. With friends like me . . . When I got out of the studio, I called the office to say: 'I think I just accidentally slagged off the UEA media team live on air.' 'Yes,' they said. 'Annie called to tell us.'

I'm not sure Annie ever forgave me, and I can't say I blame her. Had I been at UEA I would have had to cope with all sorts of competing aspects of what must have been an extremely difficult situation. My defence was that I was not at UEA. I was heading the Science Media Centre, a press office dedicated to being pro-active in the face of controversy. Asked what Professor Jones and UEA should have done in the face of this media storm there was only one answer I could give: he should have got out there and explained his emails from day one. But the reality was he couldn't do it for various reasons that I didn't have to take into account. I should have made that point in my interview, and I regret not doing so.

Two years later, in November 2011, a second batch of 5,000 stolen emails was released. This time, things were very different. When we called to ask Jones to get on a train, he did. The press briefing was packed. One by one, the journalists read out segments of emails and asked for his response. Almost all of them sounded completely different when put into context, and there were funny moments when Jones dismantled key elements of the conspiracy theory interpretation by simply explaining that activists had got the wrong year or the wrong data set – even, in one case, the wrong Mike. Jones said after the briefing: 'I wish I had been able to respond like this first time round. But until you get pushed to the edge, you never know how you'll react.' The next day the media reported it variously as 'Climategate RIP', 'The sequel that bombed', and 'Climategate II: The scientists fight back'.

Given the seriousness of the subject, I sometimes look back on the Climategate story as the biggest PR disaster ever to hit science. It was certainly one of the more prolonged. But a decade on, I am in no doubt about one thing: the science prevailed. Climate scientists didn't enjoy having to operate under a cloud of suspicion, and for far too long climate sceptics had a field day, putting the foundations of climate science under sustained assault for years. But that's exactly the point. When the dust settled after all the salvos launched against the credibility of the science, the fortress of climate science was not only unscathed – it was strengthened.

When you're in the middle of a war and feeling as if you're losing every battle, it's hard to believe that anything you're doing is making a difference. But look at where we are now in the UK: poll after poll shows that the public accepts that the climate is changing, as does every major political party and business. The arguments still rage of course, but they have moved from the science to the solutions. Those Climategate years were deeply unpleasant for Professor Phil Jones and everyone else at the sharp end. But this story vindicates our belief that scientists have everything to gain by facing controversy with a calm, clear and robust explanation of the science.

7

FROM FLOODS TO FUKUSHIMA

How to respond to breaking news

WHEN SOMETHING BIG HAPPENS like a national emergency or a major event such as disease, flooding, a rail crash or a food safety scandal – stories so big that prime ministers and other government officials must enter the fray – journalists have to move fast. With breaking news comes the risk of an information vacuum. Not all of the details will have emerged and the situation may be rapidly evolving, but in our 24/7 news era journalists have to report it instantly. The danger is that in these circumstances they may turn to sources that are easy to find rather than credible. That can lead to misrepresentations, misunderstandings, assumptions or scaremongering in the early days or hours of a big story, which can then be hard to correct further down the line. This has big implications for the public understanding of science.

Major crises share a number of features that make the circulation of misinformation more likely: politicians on all sides wading in, vying for political capital and attempting to apportion blame or offer simplistic solutions; the scale and pace of events, meaning that editors have to put general news journalists, who know less about where to go for the best experts than their specialist colleagues onto the story; and the involvement of non-governmental organisations and single-issue groups adept at seizing on crises to lobby for policy changes.

Our solution was to develop what we called 'rapid reactions' to breaking news, designed to make it easier for the media and public to hear from scientists during a fast-developing major news story. Within hours of a story breaking, journalists would open their inbox to find an SMC-curated list of the best experts available, detailed comments on aspects of the crisis and fact-checked briefing notes. Our logic was that by connecting journalists to top-quality scientists from the start of an emergency, we would make it easier for them to report accurately and ensure that there was at least evidence-based information out there among all the bluster.

Nobody else was doing this when we started. Individual universities and science organisations would contact the media if they had relevant experts, but their efforts weren't comprehensive or coordinated, nor was it necessarily a priority for overworked university media teams. There was no one-stop shop for journalists needing independent scientific commentary when a crisis broke. Here was a gap we could fill that would both improve media coverage of science and be a public good.

When a big story breaks, we drop everything else and go straight to our database. The scientists listed there have all signed up to be available to the media and have associated keywords that allow us to find the right experts for each story. We ask for an instant reaction by way of a written comment, along with an indication of their availability for interview and a willingness to engage over the coming days and weeks. These first emails are followed by further requests, for example for one-to-one interviews and specific questions from journalists as the story develops. Scientists on the lists will self-select to answer the questions that they know the most about, and agree to live interviews. Within hours, we have an efficient machine operating, with a list of scientists ready to carve out some of their time to work with us and journalists to ensure that their expertise forms part of the national discussion. That list grows as we recruit new experts in the heat of the media frenzy and it becomes an essential resource for the days, weeks or months that the story remains in the headlines. It allows the SMC to offer a 24/7 rapid-reaction service with only five press officers. Just one email, often sent out of hours from the pub or the TK Maxx changing room, is guaranteed to get the expert response the journalist needs.

Sometimes, scientists can bring knowledge to bear that stops a runaway scare story in its tracks. One of our first rapid reactions was in early January 2003, when news broke about a foiled bioterror attack on the London Underground using a chemical agent called ricin. The *Sun* reported the discovery of a 'factory of death', and the *Daily Star* claimed that '250,000 of us could have died'. We tracked down a team of ricin experts at the University of Warwick who gave us a great fact sheet on the properties of the chemical. They also told us that simply releasing the toxin into the air would probably not kill the huge number of people suggested by the press and that for ricin to be fatal it would need to be injected, swallowed or sprayed into the face and breathed in. Given access to these expert views, science journalists were able to tone down some of the scary headlines and make use of a specially compiled fact box about ricin. It was a short-lived crisis but it was also proof of concept; it showed that by acting as a conduit between journalists and scientists, the SMC could improve what the public read and heard about the science relating to a particular story.

Likewise, in 2013, when the media first revealed that horsemeat had been found in burgers and other products being sold in UK supermarkets, some journalists assumed that horsemeat was banned for health reasons and framed the story as a food safety issue. Within twenty-four hours, we had sent out comments from leading food scientists emphasising that horsemeat in itself is perfectly legal whereas omitting it from a product's list of ingredients is not. The reality was that, however culturally distasteful to us Brits, eating horsemeat does not pose a risk to health and it is actually eaten by many people across the world.

We haven't always found it easy to persuade good scientists to comment on breaking news: unlike politicians and campaigners, they are often more reluctant to respond publicly before the full facts about an incident are known. When we asked for comment on a fatal train crash or the volcanic ash crisis, I remember receiving angry emails from some scientists suggesting that they should not be expected to join the ill-informed speculation in the press. We disagreed. Of course they didn't have access to the full details of the crash in the immediate aftermath of a catastrophe – no one did. But *they* were qualified to speculate intelligently, based on their research and previous experience of similar cases. They were also much more likely to emphasise that they were speculating and to urge caution until more information was available, rather than grandstanding with overly strong claims. As we pointed out to them, for good or ill the news media will not suspend coverage until all the facts are known, so if scientists refused to do media interviews they just handed that seat in a radio studio to less-well-qualified commentators. 'If you don't do it someone else will' is a slide I show at every talk I give to scientists. The relatively new 24/7 news media is a hungry beast that needs constant feeding. We can bemoan that, or we can make sure it is being fed with good-quality evidence.

Our approach has also attracted criticism from government agencies, whose communications teams like to feel in control of the narrative, especially in the middle of a high-pressure emergency. During the media frenzy over the poisoning of Russian dissident Alexander Litvinenko in London in 2006, news reports were rife with speculation as reporters waited for details about which deadly agent had been used. First journalists talked about thallium, which they then narrowed down to radioactive thallium. The toxicologists we connected to the press emphasised that these claims about the involvement of thallium were unconfirmed, but answered media questions about the toxin's properties and what effect it might have on the human body.

One expert who found himself in particular demand was Professor John Henry, an academic specialising in toxicology at Imperial College London. He had previously worked in medicine as a consultant to the National Poisons Unit at Guy's and St Thomas' Hospital, saving the lives of many people, especially children who had ingested poisonous household products. But he had then taken the decision to move into research, exploring how poisons work and how to counteract them. He was a man who knew what he was talking about, and he undertook back-to-back interviews for us in the hours and days immediately after the attack – fielding all sorts of questions about thallium and its effects. Then the Health Protection Agency (HPA) – the predecessor to PHE – announced that the deadly agent used had in fact been polonium. Much of the information given by our experts had turned out to be irrelevant to this case, and the HPA comms team were furious, seeing what we were doing as utterly irresponsible.

We discussed their criticism a lot with our board members, scientists and journalists. The SMC was still in its infancy and we did not want to be seen as fuelling scare stories. But time and time again, we came back to the view that it was better to have experts like Henry provide informed commentary to the media than leave a vacuum to be filled by the uninformed. There are often gaps of several hours, even days, between updates from the chief medical officer or other government scientists on the latest developments. Those gaps have to be filled by someone, and generally the government scientists closest to the events are not free to do intensive media work. We have never persuaded government comms officers of our case and press officers at PHE often tell us that our rapid reactions from third-party experts are not helpful to their operations on the ground. I understand their frustrations and in an ideal world the news media would wait until facts are established before reporting. But we live very far from that ideal world and I am convinced that the public good is best served by access to good scientists at these times of national emergency.

The other thing we point out to government comms experts is that journalists often want to hear from independent scientists as well as government experts, especially during a crisis when they know that the government scientists may be subject to political pressures. I suspect journalists have often trusted official messages more *because* they have been broadly in line with what they have heard separately from independent scientists. But government communications staff like to feel in control of the narrative, especially in the middle of a high-pressure emergency, and they want the public to get clear public health messages from official sources. I like to think that someday they might recognise the value of a press office pumping out independent scientific expertise. But it seems we are not there yet.

One of the biggest emergencies we responded to before Covid was the Fukushima Daiichi incident. On Friday 11 March 2011, at 14:46 local time, there was an unprecedented undersea earthquake off the east coast of Japan. Measuring magnitude 9 on the Richter scale, it triggered a tsunami along the country's Pacific coastline, which caused immense damage and the devastating loss of almost 20,000 lives. We spent that day almost exclusively gathering comments from earth scientists, engineers and tsunami experts to send out to the press, and we left that evening hoping we'd been able to provide enough information to satisfy the media until Monday. But by Saturday morning the news broke that one of the buildings affected was a nuclear power station at Fukushima Daiichi. This was serious. The reactors had automatically shut down after the earthquake, as designed, but flooding from the tsunami had knocked out the power supply the plant needed to maintain its cooling system. If the cooling wasn't restored, the prospect of a meltdown in the reactor cores loomed. I had headed off to an annual girls' weekend away in a posh hotel in Brighton that Friday night, and was just walking into the fancy spa when I heard the news. I had to bid farewell to my girlfriends, turn around and speed back to the SMC.

On the Tuesday after the earthquake, we held an emergency briefing for journalists with experts on nuclear power and earthquakes. By this point, there had been over 5,000 confirmed casualties from the earthquake and the tsunami it had caused, and the Japanese government was already estimating that that figure would climb to over 10,000. There were as yet no confirmed deaths at Daiichi. But the nuclear power station was the only story in town for the reporters. There seems to be a peculiar fascination in the British media with stories about nuclear radiation – one reporter claims that it's because they contain an element of hidden peril that people find uniquely scary. There was also a UK angle, given that we had our own nuclear power stations and plans to build more. Questions were also being raised about whether the plume of radiation was heading our way, and whether UK citizens should be evacuated from Japan.

Thirty journalists were packed into the room, but the next day I found very few quotes in the press from our briefing. Doom-laden headlines were everywhere. One tabloid had a double-page spread with stories on 'Now Food's Nuked', 'Dangers Might Get a Lot Worse' and 'Despair of Victims in Nuke Zone'.

The next few weeks were intense as the media went into full-on catastrophe mode. Fukushima dominated the headlines, with phrases such as 'nuclear apocalypse', 'meltdown' and 'Armageddon' bandied about willy-nilly. Journalists came up with a barrage of new questions every few hours. How many millisieverts of radiation is too many? Could anything like this happen in the UK? Many talked of another Chernobyl, despite scientists repeatedly telling them that Japanese operators appeared to have done the right things to control the disaster, including setting an exclusion zone and handing out iodine tablets, which can help protect against radiation exposure. This was patently not another Chernobyl.

The experts were not downplaying the risks of the accident – many had a track record of working on nuclear safety issues or had published papers raising the alarm about previous incidents such as Chernobyl or Windscale, the UK's most serious nuclear incident back in 1957. But much of the media coverage was misleading and alarmist, and scientists were continually at pains to correct the exaggeration. Sensationalist tabloids weren't the only problem. To the general dismay of the scientific community, the EU's energy chief, Günther Oettinger, told the European Parliament: 'There is talk of an apocalypse, and I think the word is particularly well chosen.' It was hard to get calm and measured expert voices heard above the din of catastrophising, but we were determined to do it. Most science reporters joined us, fighting within their newsrooms to include more specialist commentary in their coverage.

One scientist we worked with closely throughout was Professor Paddy Regan, a nuclear physicist from the University of Surrey with a substantial track record of high-quality published research. He had good relationships with nuclear experts in Japan, and felt comfortable talking about several aspects of the story that the media were interested in. He was a clear communicator with a skill for translating highly complex nuclear physics into accessible language. Regan took to taking props to interviews, and I still remember the two white plastic beakers he would whip out to represent the reactor cores. You could often see the relief on the presenters' faces as it became clear that the nuclear physicist they had booked was a charismatic, plain-talking guy determined to help the viewers understand complex events. In an essay he wrote for us a year after Fukushima, he said of his time in the media spotlight:

> I was always impressed by the journalists who interviewed us and asked insightful questions as they got to grips with the science involved. It brought home the importance – indeed to my mind the duty – of scientists and engineers with some knowledge of esoteric topics to provide analysis and comment as events of this kind occur.

The issue of independence loomed large with Fukushima. There are certain areas of science where it is hard to find scientists who are truly independent and can be said to have no conflict of interests; nuclear power is one of them. Many experts have either worked for, or had their research funded by, industry during some part of their careers. But legitimate links with industry should not automatically rule out experts from commenting on a particular event. Those scientists with industry links that we worked with during the Fukushima crisis all had long records of publishing in established peer-reviewed journals or held positions on highly regarded scientific advisory committees. Many came from respected institutes, like the Dalton Nuclear Institute at the University of Manchester or the government-funded National Nuclear Laboratory, which necessarily collaborate with the nuclear industry as it relies on their research and expertise. Our policy is to ask every scientist to declare any and all conflicts of interest, which are then included with the comments sent to journalists. 'Let it all hang out', as we usually tell scientists, and let journalists make their own judgement. Although it's a source of some irritation to many scientists that journalists see research funding from industry as an obvious conflict but don't see any issues of bias with experts who have links to NGOs or campaign groups with clear agendas.

For some critics, the issue is less about specific financial conflicts, and more about the dangers of a kind of groupthink that could distort the way science is talked about in the media. We work regularly with many scientists on our database – potentially leading to fears that we could be promoting certain opinions more than others. This is a valid concern of course, and one we take seriously. But it would be unusual to find a scientist who has devoted his or her life to researching nuclear science who is anti-nuclear, and it does not automatically follow that a scientist who is broadly pro-nuclear cannot comment credibly on threats from particular incidents. Given how many of these scientists research safety issues, you could just as well argue that nuclear experts have a vested interest in playing up the safety risks.

None of this, however, means that we expect journalists to use the comments we offer uncritically, or that they should not include other voices in their reporting. There is rarely only one valid viewpoint when it comes to science: we tend to represent the view from mainstream science, rather than mavericks or outlying voices, but reporters should never simply leave their scepticism at the door.

In November 2011, a YouGov public opinion poll for the Nuclear Industry Association showed that public support in the UK for nuclear power, eight months after Fukushima, was almost identical to that of a year previously. Our role is not to persuade the public to take a position on nuclear power, either for or against, and we did not know precisely how public opinion had been informed by the news they heard during this crisis. But we drew comfort from the fact that people did not appear to turn against a zero-emissions source of energy as a result of the alarmist or inaccurate media reporting that did unfortunately appear. This was in sharp contrast to the reaction in other European countries, including Germany, where public opposition was so strong that Angela Merkel announced an end to Germany's nuclear programme less than three months after the incident. My theory is that the widespread debate about the pros and cons of nuclear power that followed Fukushima, improved immeasurably by the participation of good scientists, was – weirdly – the exact conversation the industry had been wanting to encourage for years. A tragic and devastating way to achieve it, but a reminder that it often takes a crisis to initiate a public discussion of science and evidence.

Two years later, I found myself sitting in Westminster at the House of Commons for the launch of an Education Media Centre modelled on the SMC. Its founding patron, former Labour education minister Baroness Morris, told how she had first heard about the SMC in the wake of the Fukushima crisis. She had noticed the large number of great scientists appearing on twenty-four-hour news channels to explain the risks of exposure to radiation, and wondered who had put them up for interview. Having learned more about radiation from these talking heads than she had ever grasped in her school science lessons, she decided that education could benefit from a similar approach.

Politics often gets in the way of reasoned discussion about causes and solutions, which I believe is even more reason to ensure that scientists are part of the media's response to breaking news. Ministers come under intense pressure to provide simple explanations and solutions to crises that are multi-faceted and complex. My colleagues and I maintain that there is a very short window at the start of a crisis – usually just a few days – when everyone seems genuinely interested in getting their heads round the facts and understanding more about the background to an issue. During those early days, the scientists we put up for press briefings and interviews are asked open-ended questions and can answer without fear of stumbling into a political row. But the window is short-lived, and we now take bets on how long it will take for politicians to start arguing about what went wrong and how to fix it. When the spats begin, it often becomes harder to persuade scientists to engage, especially if particular aspects of the crisis become the subject of a political row or a media frenzy. One story that clearly illustrates this danger is the flooding of the Somerset Levels over the winter of 2013/14.

Soon after the story broke, many non-scientists blamed the flooding on the lack of dredging of local rivers – a clear and simple explanation that naturally appealed to the media. Blaming the floods on a single contributory factor and claiming they could be prevented in future by one neat solution seemed attractive to many others too – it allowed the government to be seen taking decisive action that would yield fast results. The problem was, it wasn't true. One leading hydrologist told me that dredging might well shorten the length of time that water sits on flooded fields, but in the case of extreme flooding from a succession of heavy storms, such as this, it would probably not make much difference. In fact, in many scenarios, excessive dredging can even make flooding worse further downstream.

It was hard to make the voices of real experts heard in the ensuing media debate. Firstly, many journalists were keen on this dredging 'angle': it had simplicity, certainty and clarity – a combination beloved by journalists and arguably the public too. But also the more politicised the story became, the more reticent independent scientists felt about getting embroiled in it.

I remember attending one press briefing that was supposed to focus in part on the continued misunderstandings surrounding dredging. As the scientists arrived at the SMC, their press officer took me aside and said that various calls had taken place over the weekend and the experts had decided not to answer questions on that aspect of the crisis. I could hardly believe my ears. I appealed to them to reconsider; surely, they did not actually want me to tell a room full of journalists that they could not ask questions about the biggest element in the media coverage. To my dismay, they said they had no choice, though they looked no happier about the prospect than me. Had we had some notice, we would have pulled the briefing. Luckily there was still plenty to talk about: journalists got an in-depth briefing on the complexities and multiple causes of the flooding. But it should not be the case that independent scientists feel unable to challenge the prevailing narrative if they believe it is wrong and misleading.

I never got to the bottom of why those experts were told that dredging would have to be off the agenda for that briefing. But I've been close enough to similar situations to hazard a guess that word of the upcoming briefing had got around and calls were made from government circles to funders. As a scientist it is not easy to ignore a call from your main funder telling you not to speak about an issue. But it should worry us all that this happens. A week or so after the briefing, I woke up to the news that the government had pledged to invest millions in the dredging of rivers to prevent future flooding. While the scientists were being pressured not to give their opinions, a large sum of public money was being spent doing something that the experts knew would not solve the problem. I just can't believe that this outcome is good for anyone.

The politicisation of an issue is not the only thing that can make a scientist choose not to speak out. Sometimes, the tide of public opinion flows against scientific fact, particularly in cases with a strong human-interest angle. These can be incredibly difficult situations to navigate as they tend to be very emotionally charged, and no one wants to be unsympathetic to another's pain or seem uncaring about their plight. But when there are hard decisions to be made, we should make them based on solid, credible evidence – and to do that, we need to understand what that evidence is. Scientists should be able to speak up in such cases without fear of provoking a furious backlash. Unfortunately, this is rarely the reality, and individual scientists – as well as communications officers concerned with reputation management – can see all too clearly the downsides of being thrust into such controversial, emotive stories.

We tried desperately to get experts to speak out during the huge media coverage of the distressing end-of-life care cases of Charlie Gard and Alfie Evans, two very sick children whose parents disagreed with the medical teams treating them about whether to maintain life support. The conflicts resulted in high-profile legal battles, which dominated the media for months. Most of the clinicians with expertise on these types of issues work for NHS Trusts such as Great Ormond Street Hospital or Alder Hey Children's Hospital, and we tried hard to get them to help us with the deluge of media requests we were receiving from science and health reporters. Some were willing to speak to journalists, but told us they had been instructed not to by their hospital trusts. It was understandable, but deeply frustrating. At one stage, the Pope, Donald Trump and Theresa May had all been in the media to talk about Charlie Gard, but many of the actual experts on the subject were not allowed to speak. There were exceptions such as Professor Dominic Wilkinson, a medical ethicist from the

University of Oxford, who did weeks of back-to-back interviews for us on both occasions. But there were nowhere near enough, and health journalists struggled to reflect the views from specialist doctors in these cases, leaving the public with only a partial understanding of the wider issues involved.

The level of difficulty we encounter when recruiting scientists for our rapid reactions depends in part on the nature of the emergency. Covid was by far the worst crisis, but we had no problem lining up scientists because they could see a clear, direct connection between doing media work and encouraging the public to do what was needed to tackle infection rates. Other big stories have been more complicated, such as the Litvinenko poisoning or the 2018 Salisbury attacks, in which another former Russian agent and his daughter were exposed to the toxin Novichok (as well as a police officer and two members of the public, one of whom died). In those cases the relevant scientists were in research institutes such as the MoD's Defence Science and Technology Laboratory at Porton Down, one of the UK's most secretive research facilities, and were therefore not available to comment publicly. Emergencies such as the cloud of ash that followed the eruption of Iceland's Eyjafjallajökull volcano in 2010 have involved national security issues that made it tricky for scientists to talk to the press.

When Baroness Morris praised the public-education role played by scientists during the Fukushima crisis, it confirmed my ongoing mantra that media frenzies are an opportunity as well as a threat. The point was lost on some of the scientific bodies representing subject experts, however, when we asked them to respond to relevant breaking news stories. The comms officer of one small radiation society told us they could not put anyone up to talk about Fukushima because they were putting all their resources into a long-planned 'Radiation Week'. A similar thing happened in 2018 when the Institution of Civil Engineers refused to ask its members to comment on the Genoa bridge collapse because it was already preparing for 'Bridge Week'. These public-information campaigns, complete with hashtags and emojis, are important for small societies. But I was dismayed that they didn't see the unfortunate events in Japan and Italy as opportunities to raise awareness about radiation and bridge design respectively, during a period when people down the pub were already talking about those issues. The Fukushima crisis or 'Radiation Week' – it's not difficult to guess which made a bigger impression on the general public.

The way the media works means that attention-grabbing headlines, political rows and blame games are hard to resist, especially in times of national crisis. It will always be an uphill battle for calm, measured, expert voices to cut through the noise – but the potential benefits to the public interest in getting those expert views out there are huge. Responding rapidly to breaking news remains one of the most important things we do at the SMC, allowing policymakers and the wider public quick and easy access to people who can speak with authority about evidence, truth and facts. But such a service depends on the willingness of scientists to engage with the press – and requires a wider culture in which both scientific organisations and the media recognise the value of so doing. Too often our efforts to get scientists into the media during times of national emergency are thwarted by communications professionals who, for a variety of reasons, end up discouraging or restricting their scientists from doing media work. In a world where, for individual scientists, the benefits of speaking publicly about sometimes controversial subjects may seem nebulous at best – and dangerous at worst – that should worry us all.

8

THE SEXIST PROFESSOR?

The sorry saga of Tim Hunt

SIR TIM HUNT's very public fall from grace wasn't really a science story at all. But it was front-page news for months in the summer of 2015, and remains the biggest story about an individual scientist that I have been involved in. While many of my friends barely notice some of the stories I work on, this one was different. From my mum's elderly friends to my fellow passengers on the proverbial Clapham omnibus, everyone was talking about Tim Hunt. One of my friends, a playwright, seriously considered writing a play on it. In contrast, most of us in the scientific community soon desperately wanted it to go away.

The saga began at a lunch hosted by female Korean scientists at the World Conference of Science Journalists in Seoul, South Korea in June 2015. During his toast, Hunt was quoted as saying: 'Let me tell you about my trouble with girls. Three things happen when they are in the lab. You fall in love with them, they fall in love with you, and when you criticise them, they cry.' Not surprisingly, the words had offended some in the room.

The first I heard about it was from a former colleague attending the conference. I had run the programme committee when the conference came to London in 2009 and had loved the experience. But I've never shaken off the feeling that it is a conference that takes a rather sniffy view of science PR, and even of the type of science and health journalists we mostly work with in the UK, who have to churn out four or five science stories a day for the daily news cycle. The UK's 'science hacks' mostly don't attend. After all, which daily news outlet sends its hard-pressed journalists off to a four-day conference in exotic countries to debate their craft? For the most part, this is a conference that attracts freelance science writers, often with a formal scientific background, or science journalists working for specialist titles such as *Scientific American*, *New Scientist* or *Nature News*.

My first reaction, then, was slight bemusement as to why Tim Hunt was there at all. I didn't know him well at the time, but I had talked to his press officers at Cancer Research UK and the Royal Society in the past, and the general view was that he was a rather unworldly scientist they would generally not put in front of the camera. In that sense, he was the opposite to Sir Paul Nurse, with whom he shared the Nobel Prize in Physiology or Medicine in 2001, who is a dream with the media. That left me wondering whose bright idea it was to suggest he go to this event. My friend's texts continued into the next day, and I started to get others from more friends at the conference. Tom Feilden from BBC Radio 4 *Today* then also texted, asking if I had Hunt's mobile number. The texts from my friends in Seoul sounded unsettled, as if they didn't quite understand the way the story was developing but could sense a brewing media storm.

I woke up the next morning to find the story on the front page of *The Times* and the journalist who had tweeted his remarks was live on *Today* talking about her sense of disbelief that a leading British scientist would say such things in public.

There was a horrible inevitability about what happened in the next few hours and days. A Twitter storm was unleashed. Hunt's story became a potential new chapter for Jon Ronson's seminal book *So You've Been Publicly Shamed*, which tells the stories of individuals whose worlds came crashing down around them following an unfortunate or ill-advised tweet, joke or comment. In its initial report *Today* had managed to pre-record a reaction from Hunt at Seoul airport before he boarded his flight home. Sounding bewildered and oblivious to the media storm around him, Hunt pointed out that his comments were intended to be light-hearted and ironic. He explained that he had fallen in love with his current wife in the lab. He apologised for upsetting anyone, and sounded genuinely distressed that he had done so. But mostly he sounded as if he didn't really understand what he had done wrong. It was about the furthest you could get from the kind of slick, stage-managed apologies that we hear from politicians and celebrities with huge PR machines. Yet before he had even landed in the UK, a number of the institutions he worked for were drafting the resignation letters that they would strongly urge him to sign and send back.

Hunt's situation was a dilemma for us at the SMC. On one level, we existed to help scientists caught up in media frenzies and to provide comment on science in the headlines. Arguably, this was not really a 'science story', nor one that would have a huge impact on the public understanding of science. I was also still nervous that we did not yet have a full and accurate report of what had happened. There was contradictory information floating around about how long Hunt had spoken for and how the remarks had been received by the audience. But stepping away from a global media frenzy about a UK scientist felt wrong for the SMC, a centre now well known for running towards a media controversy rather than for the hills. Media storms wait for no man so, after several calls from scientists wanting to comment and journalists wanting to hear from them, we put out our usual call for reactive comments.

Even knowing who to approach was challenging. There was no database keyword for 'sexist professors' as there was for 'stem cells' or 'climate change'. We mostly approached the scientists we knew who had championed the role of women in science, like Professor Jackie Hunter, CEO of the Biotechnology and Biological Sciences Research Council, and Professor Dame Athene Donald at the University of Cambridge and that institution's first ever gender-equality champion. As we do for all big stories like this, we also went to the 'great and good' of science, including a number of other vice-chancellors and many CEOs and presidents of research institutes and Royal Colleges. The ten comments we issued over the next twenty-four hours all condemned Hunt's remarks. Jackie Hunter summed up the general mood when she said: 'We have a long way to go in tackling unconscious bias in science, especially at senior levels, but these [damaging] remarks show that even conscious bias still exists.'

I understood the anger from Hunter and others. Hunt's flippant remarks echoed the sexist attitudes of some eminent male scientists they had encountered in their own careers, and which had no doubt led to many promising young female scientists deciding against a career in the lab.

While I was busy arranging broadcast interviews with the scientists who had provided us with comments, we became aware of two interesting things. Firstly, there was a noticeable difference in response between the female scientists we approached who knew Hunt and those who did not. The former group insisted that he was not sexist. Those who did not know him were furious. Secondly, I was getting calls from senior scientists and institutions asking me to help Hunt. His bewildered performance on the *Today* programme had convinced many of his friends and colleagues that he needed media support from an experienced press officer. Several of the calls came from people whose press officers felt unable to support Hunt openly because they were busy drafting comments distancing themselves from him or, worse, drafting his resignation letter.

I called Hunt later that same day, catching him as he waited to collect his luggage at Heathrow. The first thing I asked was whether he knew how serious this was. He brushed it off, saying he knew he had said something stupid but did not believe he was in trouble. I changed tack. 'Tim, are you listening to me? Trust me. You are in trouble. Big trouble.' What a welcome home!

By the time we met the next day, less than seventy-two hours after he had made his remarks, Hunt had already been sacked from an honorary position at University College London (UCL) and a Royal Society prize-giving committee, and within another day would be sacked from the board of the European Research Council (ERC). Or, rather, his 'resignation had been accepted' by these institutions. There wasn't much I could do at that point. The idea of getting Hunt to tour broadcast studios, as Professor David Nutt had done when he found himself at the heart of a media storm (see Chapter 5), did not feel like the right option for him. Nor was I warming to the suggestion made by several of his friends of drafting a slicker, more rehearsed apology for him. I've always disliked inauthentic apologies that look as though they were written by some faceless crisis comms agency, and I suspect the public sees right through them. It was also clear to me that no apology would be strong enough for some people in any case. They wanted his head on a plate.

By now, journalists had learnt that I was in touch with Hunt and had started lobbying me to pass on their requests for interviews. When critics later suggested I was secretly advising him, I could at least smile at the idea that it was secret: he had arrived for our first meeting at the SMC just as all of the UK's main science journalists were spilling out of a packed briefing room. It was also interesting to see how some science journalists who were attacking the academic on Twitter were then calling me, promising to be delightful to him if I got them an interview.

One request I remember from a major broadcaster came with the pre-condition that Hunt would have to demonstrate both in advance of and during the interview 'that he gets it. I mean really Gets It.' I asked exactly what that meant, and they answered that he would need to show that he understood the damage and harm he had done to all women in science, and that he understood that he represented everything that was wrong with science today. The truth as I saw it was that Hunt did not 'get' that. Any of it. In my early chats with him, it was clear that he had no clue what was happening to him and no frame of reference to help him grasp it. I lived full-time in the land of media frenzies, Twitter storms and science controversies. Hunt's world was about cancer research and inspiring the next generation of European scientists. In our very first meeting, he started by pulling out his laptop to show me, not something related to the conference or his remarks, but a mass of impenetrable data and graphs from a new cancer research paper he was excited about. Hunt was just not interested in news – his radio was tuned to BBC Radio 3, for God's sake.

The more time I spent with him, the more I became convinced that broadcast interviews would be disastrous for Hunt. Not because he was a sexist pig, but because he just could not fully engage with what was happening to him or articulate a cogent response. Despite reports to the contrary, Hunt never tried to explain away his comments or defend them. He never mentioned to me that he might have said anything else that might cast his remarks in a different light; it was other journalists who would later reveal that his toast had been reported selectively. While others obsessed endlessly over who said what when, Hunt never showed the slightest interest.

When we first met, I asked Hunt to explain exactly what had happened at the conference. He told me that he had delivered his keynote lecture, the reason he was there, directly before the ill-fated toast. He explained that it had not gone to plan because a technical problem resulted in a mix up with his slides. The problem was finally sorted out, but Hunt said that he had rushed to the sponsored lunch feeling flustered and upset because he had not been able to deliver the best version of his lecture. He was also missing Massimo Gaudina, his good friend and media adviser at the ERC, who had arranged for him to attend this conference and was due to accompany him, but had had to back out at the last minute. Finally, and this was why Hunt had been so adamant that there was not a problem when I spoke to him at the airport, he claimed that no one in the room had challenged him at the time or immediately after his toast, and the journalists who reported his comments on Twitter had not approached him for reaction. A US journalist he knew did raise the topic over breakfast the following morning, but Hunt remembered that conversation as a kindly rebuke rather than a confrontation.

The first bid I received for Hunt from a print journalist came from Robin McKie at the *Observer*. McKie had been the paper's science editor for over thirty years and had reported on Hunt's research many times before. He stressed that, if Hunt revealed sexist attitudes or repeated any sexist comments, he would obviously report them, and he wanted us to know that this interview was not going to be cosy or risk-free. That was fine by me. I knew McKie would give him a fair hearing.

At first, Hunt said no to the interview. I had decided that I would pass each request to him, offer my advice and then let him make his own decisions. I was offering support I felt he needed, but I was not his official press officer and I encouraged him to ask other press officers he knew for their thoughts too. I was also still unsure whether conducting media interviews was the right option on this occasion. This view was at odds with everything I usually stand for. I am always the advocate in science for speaking out, whatever the risks and sensitivities. But in prior cases such as climate change and animal research, there was a public interest in hearing from experts and it was important for scientists to challenge misleading information about their work. In this case, the only question about misleading information related to Hunt, not his work. It wasn't my job to save his reputation, but I definitely did not want to offer advice that made things worse for him either.

Given that Hunt seemed unwilling or unable to mount his own defence, the risks of any interviews outweighed the rather nebulous benefits. Set against that, I knew that some of the pressure might ease if he did at least one interview with a widely respected science journalist, and I wanted people to hear his authentic voice. I made these points to him and he reluctantly agreed. McKie agreed to let me go with him to the interview and we travelled together to the cottage in rural Hertfordshire that Hunt shared with his wife, UCL academic Professor Mary Collins.

I suspect crisis comms agencies would be gobsmacked that I did not prepare 'lines' for Hunt for that interview – or, indeed, do any preparation at all. Many will think that was wholly irresponsible, and they may be right. But I knew in my waters that slick crisis comms PR was not right for someone like Hunt. It wasn't my strong suit either, and certainly would not win over Robin McKie – a fan of substance and science over style. And by now, I was forming the strong view that this scientist was popular with so many for good reason. I felt there was a good chance he would come over sympathetically without any coaching from anyone.

I had told Hunt that McKie would love to hear from Professor Collins too – and I was personally intrigued as to whether she might defend or condemn him. I had nothing but sympathy for this woman who, through no fault of her own, had woken up in the middle of a global media storm around sexism in science – something she had challenged all her working life. Initially, she said no, but by the time we arrived she had decided to go on the record, and it was her painful cry that they had both been hung out to dry that grabbed the headline. Collins was visibly distressed and spent much of the interview with her head in her hands. 'It was an unbelievably stupid thing to say,' she acknowledged candidly, adding that his language was sometimes stuck firmly in the past. 'I am a feminist, and I would not have put up with him if he were sexist.' She described the moment when her husband received the call from the ERC, which he had helped to set up, asking him to resign, saying that they both simply sat together and cried.

By then I didn't need much more persuading that Tim Hunt was the wrong poster boy for sexism in science, and I went on the record with that view. Some suggested I was too quick to draw that conclusion but, as I pointed out, I took several days longer to arrive at my conclusion than it took many commentators to decide the opposite. And unlike others, perhaps, I had made about ten calls to women I knew who had worked closely with Hunt, all of whom confirmed what I was now hearing from multiple sources – that he was incredibly generous with his time in mentoring young students, irrespective of gender. His investment in these students arguably made a material difference to their careers.

I knew that Hunt's remarks were sexist, and I also knew that many women's careers had been blighted by sexist attitudes in labs. But the widespread assumption that his comments meant that he must have frequently hindered his female colleagues increasingly struck me as spectacularly unfair. I felt someone needed to say that out loud. Prominent female scientists who had spent their lives battling against sexist attitudes in science, including

Professor Dame Ottoline Leyser and Professor Dame Valerie Beral, had worked closely with Hunt at some point in their careers. They did not defend his comments, but they were upset about what they saw as a hasty rush to judgement on his overall character. Nor was there necessarily a generational divide. I was contacted by Dr Alessia Errico, a young Spanish researcher in one of Hunt's labs who was desperate to go public with her experience of his generous mentoring of her and other female students in the lab. I suggested she approach *Nature*, which published her account of the six years she had enjoyed working in his lab and his inspiring support. Describing how Hunt had persuaded her to present their joint research at scientific meetings in front of eminent audiences, she wrote:

> I have seen discrimination and sexism in science and in wider society. I have seen female colleagues talked about in negative ways when they left the lab to have children. The issue is a genuine one that demands urgent attention. But it is grossly unfair that Tim should be considered, and treated, as an emblem of this sexism or gender discrimination.

She concluded that, alongside female role models in science, we also need inspirational figures.

Despite huge media scrutiny and a desperate search for more examples of Hunt's sexism, the accounts that were emerging painted a picture of a far kinder and more generous figure than the sexist ogre initially depicted. His ex-wife gave an interview to the *Daily Mail* in which she described herself as a strident feminist and said, 'I won't say anything against him'. Others told of how he had fought a successful campaign to have a nursery established at the Okinawa Institute of Science and Technology and had tried to do the same (albeit unsuccessfully) at the Francis Crick Institute – things Hunt, characteristically, never thought of bringing up himself.

Even those furiously distancing themselves from the academic were privately telling me how much they regretted having to do so. Imran Khan, then CEO of the British Science Association, provided us with a comment condemning Hunt's remarks, but told me he was really sorry to have to ask him to stand down from judging their Young Scientist of the Year campaign because he had been one of the best judges and the most generous with his time. A friend at the Nobel Foundation was virtually in tears as she described his humility and generosity in mentoring young scientists, noting how different he was to many more egotistical winners.

The Royal Society stopped short of removing his Fellowship but, under intense pressure to be seen to take some action, asked him to resign from one of its prize-giving committees. Of course, the 'resignation' then hit the headlines. When I quizzed senior staff about whether they believed Hunt had or would allow any sexist views to cloud his judging, they said they did not. But the society took the view that by publicly describing himself as a chauvinist, as he had in his ill-fated remarks, he had made it impossible for it not to act. The same could be said of the sacking by the ERC. Everyone I spoke to there, including the president, scientists on the Council and communications staff, wanted to stand by Hunt. The ERC staff member who had been with him at the lunch had made verbatim notes on his talk and had circulated a confidential report internally, which was clearly at odds with elements of the version circulating around the globe. However, senior officials from the European Commission disregarded the ERC's supposedly independent Scientific Council and its president and asked Hunt to resign.

At that time, Hunt was dedicating much of his life to the ERC, including travelling a lot to spread the word about the benefits of European science. In a very real sense, he was working for them: he was booked up for years ahead. But like many eminent scientists with multiple hats, Hunt held many honorary fellowships, including one at UCL. He was never actually employed by the university, yet UCL was the first institution to go public on ceasing its association with him, a story that became headline news throughout the national and global media. Many senior scientists at UCL wanted tough action, feeling that being the first to act against Hunt would send a strong message about UCL's commitment to women in science. It didn't necessarily play out that way, though, as others reacted against what they saw as an unseemly haste to pass judgement and a lack of due process. In the interview with the *Observer*, Professor Collins, herself a senior scientist at UCL, revealed that her husband had been sacked by way of a call she received from a senior UCL colleague while Hunt was still mid-flight from Korea. This colleague had said that, if Hunt didn't resign as soon as he landed, he would be dismissed. (No one except the science press officers in UCL pointed out that he had no job to either resign or be sacked from, and that there was therefore no need to issue any statement or get involved in the story at all.) As a senior scientist at UCL, Professor Collins was inevitably caught in the crossfire between her employer and her husband. I sensed that she was more affected by the situation than him. Hunt's unworldliness somehow gave him more scope for escape. Professor Collins, by contrast, was more firmly rooted in the real world of science and understandably felt as if it had abandoned her.

I am not sure why the tide turned towards Tim Hunt in the media, but turn it did. *The Times* was the paper that first covered the story and brought it to the world's attention. But within a week, the paper was running leader articles backing Hunt and lambasting the organisations that had turned their backs on him, claiming they 'should be more embarrassed than he is'. One journalist told me the change of heart came after the newspaper's editor was berated by friends at a dinner party. The paper subsequently became Hunt's chief cheerleader. Well-known figures in science, including Brian Cox and Richard Dawkins, were invited by *The Times* to support Hunt and enthusiastically agreed. When they had exhausted their list of famous scientists, the paper turned to other high-profile UCL alumni such as David Dimbleby, who resigned his own honorary fellowship in protest. *The Times* followed every twist and turn of the story over the next six months.

In time, the battle lines were clearly drawn. The *Daily Mail* joined *The Times* in backing Hunt, while the *Guardian* ran an editorial defending UCL:

> The Hunt camp claims feminists are too humourless to see that it was a joke. But as the provost of UCL, Professor Michael Arthur, pointed out when he indicated last Friday that Professor Hunt would not be reinstated, it was impossible for an institution to tolerate someone to whom they had awarded an honorary post, even a 72-year-old Nobel prize winner, expressing views even in jest that so comprehensively undermined its own reputation as a leading supporter of female scientists.

Lobbied by many female scientists who were increasingly frustrated by the narrow and partisan nature of the debate, I tried, and occasionally succeeded, in placing comment pieces that attempted to move the focus away from one individual to the broader issues facing women in science. There were some attempts, including by BBC Radio 4's *Women's Hour*, to grapple with systemic and structural issues. But mostly it was a battle between self-declared Hunt supporters and critics, played out in rival papers with the man himself nowhere to be seen. In perhaps the most bizarre aspect of this saga, *Sun* columnist and former MP Louise Mensch and author Dan Waddell took opposing sides in an extraordinary feud over the issue, devoting tens of thousands of words to proving each other wrong in their interpretation of what had happened.

Somehow, this sorry saga dragged on for months. I was grateful for the occasional flash of levity, such as my conversations with the reluctant reporter put on the story by *The Times*. Tom Whipple is a smart, affable journalist who loves nothing more than a quirky story about chimpanzees' sexual practices or problem-solving crows. Yet for six months of his life he was effectively chief Tim Hunt reporter, scrabbling around for ways to keep the story going on the instructions of his editor. I once found him skulking in a corner at the Royal Society's sought-after annual summer soiree, having been told to spend the evening getting yet more famous scientists to side with Hunt, and amusing rumours swirled that he had been forcibly ejected from the top-secret UCL council meeting discussing the university's actions.

One of the few significant revelations that emerged after the original story broke was that Hunt's supposedly thirty-seven-word toast was actually twice as long as had been initially reported. The full version, as reported verbatim by an EU official present at the talk, was leaked to *The Times* two weeks into the fallout. It read like this:

It's strange that such a chauvinist monster like me has been asked to speak to women scientists. Let me tell you about my trouble with girls. Three things happen when they are in the lab: you fall in love with them, they fall in love with you, and when you criticise them, they cry. Perhaps we should make separate labs for boys and girls? Now seriously, I'm impressed by the economic development of Korea. And women scientists played, without doubt, an important role in it. Science needs women and you should do science despite all the obstacles, and despite monsters like me.

A follow-up article revealed that the EU official also said Hunt's remarks were well received, contradicting his accusers' claims of an uncomfortable silence (or even a 'deathly silence' as one described it on Radio 4) and that one of the luncheon's organisers, a woman from the Korean National Research Council of Science and Technology, told him 'she was impressed that Sir Tim could improvise such a warm and funny speech'.

In the days that followed, this account was corroborated by several people who had attended the luncheon. One of them, Russian science journalist Natalia Demina, had challenged the accusations against Hunt from the very start on Twitter.

I was far less excited about these revelations than some of Hunt's supporters, who argued they showed that, while clumsily expressed, the target of his remarks was meant to be himself rather than women scientists. By this stage, most people had made up their minds about Hunt and those who felt he deserved his fate were unlikely to be persuaded otherwise. For many, his remarks were inexcusable and damaging irrespective of his intent or any wider context. I had no wish to persuade them otherwise: for me, the significance of this revelation lay more in the reliability of the original reporting on the affair, which seemed somewhat selective.

In recent years, I have often reflected on whether we were right to advise and support Hunt. Just as in the outside world, at the time there were differing views within the SMC's board: some members thought I was far too sympathetic to the academic, while others asked me to do more to support him. Professor Chris Chambers, a scientist at Cardiff University who was a member of our advisory committee at the time, passionately disagreed with me on the subject, and we had a lengthy and intense email debate that went on for weeks. My chairman Jonathan Baker expressed concern over whether we had the right skills to properly support Hunt. And another of our advisory committee members, Fay Schlesinger from *The Times*, wished I had offered Hunt's exclusive to her paper rather than the *Observer*. For my part, I am still not sure. It was such an unusual situation that it's hard to draw any hard and fast conclusions. While my personal sympathies publicly lay with Hunt, by far the greater part of the SMC's involvement with this story was in issuing quotes, setting up interviews and placing op-eds from senior female scientists who were deeply angered by his words and wanted to use the row to draw attention to the barriers facing women in science.

What to make of this media story then? Certainly it is hard to see that any winners emerged from what still feels a little like a Shakespearean tragedy. If there are any lessons to be learned – and I am not entirely sure there are – I would argue that, in the age of global social media, science press officers should use the Tim Hunt affair to reflect on the right balance between the need to respond quickly, the duty of care they owe to any figures involved, and the importance of establishing the facts as early as possible. As Mike Granatt, senior partner at Luther Pendragon and former head of the Government Communication Service, said to me:

> Importantly, the best press officers agree that a rush to recognition is an essential demonstration of awareness

and engagement. But they know that a rush to judgement with limited knowledge is a trap, all too easily sprung by campaigners or happenstance or both. They need to stand their ground.

Perhaps institutions should decide now on some ground rules for similar cases in future, to avoid being similarly overwhelmed by events. If so, I would propose this: that no scientific body should make any significant decisions about its association with a scientist based primarily on reports in the national news or social media.

***

The SMC holds a Christmas party each year for which we send out an invitation that pokes fun at some of the big science stories of the year. That year we told guests that the dress code was 'distractingly sexy', a reference to the hashtag that went viral on social media in the wake of the Hunt affair. Using this hashtag, female scientists took to posting images of themselves as they actually appeared at work – dressed variously in lab coats, goggles, helmets and full-body biohazard suits. We invited Hunt and Professor Collins to the party, assuring the couple that they would be perfectly safe, even in a room of journalists. They accepted the invitation but before the party got properly started, they told me they were leaving the UK: Collins had taken a senior role at the Okinawa Institute of Science and Technology. The loss of such an accomplished female academic to UK science was just one of the horrible ironies of this saga. Early the next morning, I took a call from a journalist asking if the rumour flying around the party was true – were the couple leaving the UK? Not so safe after all. I apologised to Hunt, but he was sanguine. Being in the news for heading to Japan was something he could handle.

When I blogged about the Tim Hunt saga at the time, I wrote that although the ivory tower of science might still feel closed to many women, adorning its gates with the head of Dr Hunt did nothing for equality. I still feel that way six years later. If those people who sacked him or called for his resignation ever felt this was a victory, it was surely a pyrrhic one. The UK has lost one of its most senior female scientists – together with one of its most inspirational.

9

STRANGE BEDFELLOWS

The uneasy relationship between scientists and science journalists

WHILE PREPARING TO INTERVIEW for the role of head of the newly planned SMC, I had seen accounts from many scientists who believed that the media coverage on issues such as MMR and GM had undermined public trust in science. But when I undertook a closer reading of science stories written at that time, I discovered a mixed picture. Many of the sensationalist stories had been written by general reporters, political hacks and consumer journalists feeding off media-savvy campaigners rather than good scientists. The coverage provided by science journalists was mostly well balanced. During the consultation process we held in our first few months, I spoke to a number of great science journalists who were generous with their time and indulged my endless questions about what value a new press office for science could add. What became clear was that there was little I could teach them about good science reporting, but they were as frustrated as the scientists about the sensationalist coverage of issues such as cloning, nuclear energy and mobile phones. Our discussions focused on how the SMC could help improve things by encouraging scientists to engage with them and by enhancing the status of the science specialist within the newsroom.

Some have speculated that science reporters are a particular breed of journalist. Fran Unsworth, former head of news at the BBC, was once asked why so few senior managers at the corporation had come from a science reporting background. She hesitated briefly before saying that the science journalists at the BBC tended to love their jobs and prefer reporting to management. It was something I had noticed beyond the BBC too: many science, health and environment reporters had done more than twenty years on the beat. When asked why he loves science reporting, Tom Feilden said:

> It's almost always exploratory rather than accusatory – so both me and the scientists go home happy! And then what a privilege it is – a licence to poke around in the labs of some of the brightest people on the planet asking impertinent questions about their life's work. Then there's the variety . . . biomedical science, space, climate, biodiversity, palaeontology . . . Finally, it matters. Science is integral to a modern society.

When debating why there was such tension between science and the media at the time the SMC opened in 2002, there was talk of a clash between the values of science and news. The late Professor Sir Richard Doll, the scientist who discovered the link between smoking and cancer, once described it like this to a room of journalists: 'You don't like harping on about things that have been public knowledge for some time. You like things that are new. But unfortunately things that are new in science are often wrong, whereas things that are true take time to build up.'

More reflective journalists, meanwhile, are often brutally honest about the limits of truth telling in the media. David Broder, a long-serving journalist at the *Washington Post*, said back in 1979: 'I would like to see us say – over and over again, until the point has been made – that the newspaper that drops on your doorstep is a partial, hasty, incomplete, inevitably somewhat flawed and inaccurate rendering of some of the things we have heard about in the past twenty-four hours.' Not surprising, then, that scientists are wary of journalists and journalists find it challenging to work with scientists. I can well remember seeing the horror on the faces of a room of Royal Society Fellows when a broadsheet editor told them that, in his newsroom, there would only be one answer to the question: 'Do you want it now, or do you want it correct?'

I started my media relations career with a journalism degree, and still remember the lecture where an ex-journalist told us 'Car crash – no one dead' will never be a story. 'Car crash – five teenagers dead' is what will get people's attention. Media-studies students have debated these news values for decades, and there have been many bold attempts to do things differently. We have, for example, seen the emergence of 'slow news' outlets such as *Tortoise Media*, which aspire to offer an alternative to the faster-is-better model by producing 'slow journalism' that takes the time to report the bigger, more complicated news in more depth over a longer period. But, while plenty has changed in the media land-scape, traditional news values have proved remarkably resilient.

Everything we do at the SMC is intended to support high standards in science reporting. But we saw an extra opportunity to try to influence those standards in 2011 during the Leveson Inquiry, an investigation by Lord Justice Brian Leveson into the practices of the UK media following the News International phone hacking scandal. It was my then colleague Helen Jamison who suggested we submit evidence to the inquiry. After a few glasses of what she calls 'lady petrol', and with her Mancunian accent coming out after a drink, she declared: 'It's not hacking celebrities' phones that harms the public interest – it's shit science coverage.' The next day, we emailed several science press officers asking what issues they would highlight, and within a week we had submitted pages of written evidence.

When I later told my colleagues I had been called to give oral evidence, they thought it was a wind-up. We had been obsessively following coverage of the inquiry for weeks on the main bulletins, lapping up appearances by high-profile media figures such as Rebekah Brooks, Alastair Campbell, Paul Dacre and Andy Coulson. And now me. It was exciting and daunting in equal measure – I was the only person from the science community who had been called to appear, so I felt I had to get this right.

I had never been in a courtroom before, though, and my nerves were plainly visible. My abiding memory is of Robert Jay QC and Lord Justice Leveson himself repeatedly pleading with me to slow down. The official transcript shows that after failing with his first two attempts, Leveson said: 'Don't feel you have to speak quickly because it's only half an hour. I can extend the time . . . I'm just concerned that smoke seems to be emanating from the shorthand writer.'

The main thing I wanted to get across was the media's attachment to its longstanding values, as I'd described them in my written evidence:

> The appetite for a great scare story; the desire to overstate a claim made by one expert in a single small study; the reluctance to put one alarming piece of research into its wider, more reassuring context; journalistic balance which conveys a scientific divide where there is none; the love of the outlier; and so on.

Helpfully, that day's *Independent* served to reinforce my point with a two-page splash headlined: 'Once they were blind, now they see

– patients cured by stem cell "miracle". Except, they hadn't been cured. Although the patients had reported a slight improvement (they had poor vision and were registered blind), this was just a safety study and had involved only two patients. Of course, it was worth reporting – it was a significant development at a time when stem cell research was in its infancy and trials using real people were only just beginning – but the way it was reported suggested the science was much further along, and it could have given false hope to thousands of people with macular degeneration.

It was with huge trepidation later that day that I called Steve Connor, science editor on the *Independent*, to tip him off that I had held up his work at the Leveson Inquiry as an example of poor science reporting. I can't exactly say he was thrilled but, to my relief, he was at least sanguine. The report he had filed the night before had been much more nuanced, but the night editors had decided to make it the day's 'splash' and the sub-editors had got to work on the headline. Connor sent me the original piece he had filed, and we played 'spot the difference' in the office.

As I was leaving the courtroom, I was stopped by the managing editor of the *Sun*. As part of my evidence, I had also been disparaging about a scare story it had run a week earlier about chemicals in household products under the headline 'Breast cancer "risk" all over shops' shelves', so I assumed he was going to take issue with me. Instead, he said that the paper really wanted to get the science right in its coverage and asked if we would go in and do a session on science reporting for the general news journalists. As the Leveson Inquiry rolled on, it felt as if a change in the standards of reporting was finally happening – and that it was going to include science coverage.

While giving evidence, I had asserted the need for a new set of guidelines for science reporting, which I had boldly claimed would only take a few hours for us to draft alongside journalists and scientists. In fact, when the inquiry called a week later asking us to go ahead, it turned into a tortuous day-long drafting session. At a couple of stages, I thought we might not get it done at all, especially when it came to the thorny issue of headlines. The journalists and sub-editors insisted that headlines need to be eye-catching and pithy rather than an accurate summary of what lies beneath. The scientists in the room were outraged, seeing this as a licence to be inaccurate. I felt like one of those negotiators in global peace talks, who has to keep everyone in the room somehow in order to get the deal. But there was a mutual determination to make it work, and we eventually came up with a compromise: headlines should not mislead the reader about a story's contents, and quotation marks should not be used to dress up overstatements.

Overall, the new guidelines were intended to encourage journalists to report science in a way that helps the public understand which evidence is reliable, and which is still a work in progress. Some of the guidelines, for example, read: state the source of the story so readers can look it up; specify the size, nature and limitations of the study; and indicate the stage of the research and a realistic time-frame for any new treatment or technology to reach the public.

We sent the guidelines to Lord Justice Leveson and, to our delight, he recommended them in his final report. The Independent Press Standards Organisation – set up in the aftermath of the Leveson Inquiry – now promotes them in newsrooms, and the fact that editors and journalists were involved in drawing them up means that we've seen them more readily embraced than might otherwise have been the case.

When giving talks to scientists, I show them examples of news stories that are more measured and accurate because scientists got involved. One I like to show from the *Daily Mail* back in 2008, was reporting on a study in mice showing a link between a commonly used moisturiser and cancer. The reporter, Fiona MacRae, included comments from two different experts questioning the relevance of the research to human skin and pointing out the study would need replicating in humans. One of the experts said that it would be 'crazy' to stop using moisturisers based on the research, adding: 'Studies of mouse skin cancer have contributed little to our understanding of human skin cancer.' The best bit was the headline, which read: 'Skin cancer link to moisturiser (but only in mice)', with the caveat in the same large font as the main claim. It shows how a good journalist can tell an interesting story while making sure readers know it's too early to stop slapping on the face cream. In these talks, I also deliberately pepper my slides with examples from the tabloids to challenge the prejudices of academics. Whatever you think of the *Mail*'s editorial lines, their science reporting is generally good, especially when they are not in campaign mode, and sometimes better than the broadsheets. I also like to point out that the *Mail* is the second-biggest-selling newspaper in the UK and that, when combined with its online audience, it attracts a readership far larger than any of the broadsheets. In a very real sense, if scientists want to better inform the public, they absolutely should talk to the *Daily Mail*.

But for every well-balanced article, there are plenty more that misrepresent the science. One person who has had great success in drawing this to people's attention is Dr Ben Goldacre, who burst on to the scene in 2003 as the 'Bad Science' columnist for the *Guardian*'s new science supplement, and went on to write a bestselling book of the same name. We all revelled in his weekly takedowns of quacks, dodgy nutritionists and the tabloids' latest 'Cure for Alzheimer's'. The downside, however, of a weekly column called 'Bad Science' is that it is necessarily selective, and risks creating a partial and therefore distorted perspective on science reporting. The *Independent*'s Jeremy Laurance reflected the exasperation of many science journalists when he lashed out at Goldacre for a column criticising one too many health reporters:

> Is Ben Goldacre, the celebrated author of *Bad Science* and scourge of health journalists everywhere, losing it? So accustomed has he become to swinging his fists at the media when they get a science story wrong, I fear he may one day go nuclear and take out three rows of medical correspondents with a single lungful of biting sarcasm.

Goldacre was a powerful force for good in newsrooms for years, with journalists telling me that they warned their news editors to avoid running certain stories or risk being 'Goldacred' in Saturday's *Guardian*. Dr Richard Horton, editor of the *Lancet*, once pressed Goldacre to spell out how he would fix the problem. He answered that we should stop reporting science as news and, instead, write developments up as longer features when the evidence has built to the extent that it's established and reliable. I have some sympathy for this view, and I know many scientists share it. Far too many daily reports are from early and preliminary studies publicised too soon; small studies that still need to be reproduced on a larger scale; or an observational study, which can suggest X might be linked to Y, but cannot prove a causal link. Many of these are assigned far too much prominence, given that they will never come to anything. But we must remember how hugely significant it is that science has finally taken its place alongside politics, education and economics as a core news subject. Science is too important to be annexed and separated from daily news. The SMC's approach is to get the science in the news reported in a more measured way rather than to confine it to long-form journalism (though both would be nice).

There was a collective sigh of relief from the metaphorical Fleet Street when Goldacre moved from calling out 'bad science' to 'bad pharma', advocating for openness in clinical research. In his final column, he reflected on the challenges of changing mainstream media, adding: 'It's worth it, for one simple reason: pulling bad science apart is the best teaching gimmick I know for explaining how good science works.' His book is testament to that and remains one of the best 'explainers' on the scientific method I know. During Covid, he was one of the lead authors on OpenSAFELY, a research platform that used GP records to identify those most at risk of catching the virus. Presenting his results at several SMC briefings, it was nice to see him actively helping journalists to avoid the pitfalls he had called them out on for years.

In his book *Flat Earth News*, Nick Davies argues that journalists themselves are not the reason for the increase in 'falsehood, distortion and propaganda' that we have seen across the media world. Instead, the problem is structural, with fewer journalists having to fill more and more space in our new 24/7 news cycle. Davies argues this leads to 'churnalism', where even good journalists end up regurgitating press releases with no time to check facts or ask critical questions. Science journalism is not immune from this trend. In the past, most publications and broadcasters were happy with a handful of stories a week, and many of those were assigned as the lightweight, quirky 'and finally' story at the end of the evening news. Increasingly now, science stories are as likely to be headline news as politics or economics, from missions to Mars to climate change to genome editing. This is cause for celebration, but the media's insatiable appetite for science news has brought challenges.

Tim Radford, former *Guardian* science editor, has often waxed lyrical about his early days as a science journalist, travelling the country visiting labs, meeting incredible scientists, and unearthing original stories. But that was when journalists had the luxury of time; now, they are expected to deliver four or five stories a day, if not more. Of course, that leaves less time for fact-checking, original reporting, and seeking out third-party comments. It also has implications for the quality of the journalism: it is simply not always possible to maintain the highest standards of reporting under such conditions.

At the SMC, we worked out early on that we could either bemoan this state of affairs and sit in judgement or we could work out ways to support journalists to report well despite these pressures. The SMC's work is designed to make it easier for time-poor news journalists to find the credible, accurate information and the scientists they need to write measured stories. Critically, the starting point for our work is what news journalists need. There is zero point in sending out information if it's not in a form that they can easily use in their reporting.

Our approach has attracted some criticism, primarily from journalism academics or science writers who work outside the daily news cycle. There tend to be three main lines of argument, as helpfully outlined by one vocal critic, Connie St Louis, a former science journalist who taught science journalism at City, University of London. The first is that our model reinforces negative developments such as the 'churnalism' identified by Nick Davies. The second is that our practice of sending out expert quotes to journalists (often described pejoratively as 'canned quotes' by critics) means that journalists are in effect putting the responsibility to scrutinise scientific claims into our hands, which is less likely to lead to original and critical reporting. Lastly, St Louis has argued that the SMC has become too powerful, with our choice of topics and scientists having too much influence over what appears in the news.

I think such criticism is helpful. We share many of our critics' concerns about the pressures on journalists today and how they can affect the quality of journalism. In particular, we recognise that the services we offer to the news media *are* a de facto acceptance of the way things are in journalism rather than an attempt to change them. But our remit is to get better science into the media, not to overhaul journalism itself. Our creation may have been symptomatic of the decline of the kind of independent, critical reporting that journalism academics champion, but we are certainly not the cause. In fact, our job often includes working closely with journalists on exclusive investigations or tipping off journalists: in 2020, when a leading scientist decided to turn whistle-blower on a story about scientific fraud, we took the story to Ian Sample at the *Guardian*, knowing he would do justice to it.

I do hate the phrase 'canned quotes', though. This derogatory description of one aspect of our work spectacularly misses the point. Of course some hard-pressed journalists with thousands of words to file will use a quote from a credible source if they feel it's relevant – and why not? But 'canned' suggests some kind of vacuous, pre-prepared statement, which could not be further from the truth. Each comment we issue on a new study is produced by the scientist after reading that particular study. If we suspect that they haven't read the paper, we will push back, asking them to read the text in full and provide more detail. Often the comments we collect are detailed explanations of highly technical issues. Nor are they always simply copied. Broadcasters use them to identify potential guests, while print journalists will read them before putting in a call to the scientist to ask them to elaborate further. Journalists can scan them quickly to see where the weight of scientific opinion lies, and whether scientists are mostly agreed on something or divided. They can also use them to help assess whether a new study is significant or not. The late Nigel Hawkes, former health editor and science editor of *The Times*, once said he had come to trust SMC third-party comments on new research so much that he often read them before reading a journal press release and paper to help decide whether to report it.

Criticism of what we do has afforded us some great opportunities to engage in critical debate about our work, including a major profile on me in *Nature* for the tenth anniversary of the SMC. Reporter Ewen Callaway spent several weeks shadowing me, interviewing colleagues and talking to critics. The article opened: 'Depending on whom you ask, Fiona Fox is either saving science journalism or destroying it.' The *Nature* photographer assigned to the piece admitted she hadn't shot any non-scientists for the publication before. Maybe that's why she thought it would be a good idea to have me pose with my stiletto on top of a pile of newspapers that she'd painstakingly arranged for the purpose. I refused point blank – clearly she hadn't quite got what the SMC was all about.

One of the SMC's catch phrases is 'the media will do science better when scientists do the media better'. But of course sometimes even the most media-friendly scientists discover that being a good journalist involves particular skills that scientists don't possess. Professor Sir David Spiegelhalter, Professor of the Public Understanding of Risk at the University of Cambridge, has been a hugely influential voice on science and the media, regularly appearing on TV and radio to put into context terrifying headlines about the risks of everything from a bacon sandwich to a glass of wine. Justin Webb, presenter on BBC Radio 4's *Today* programme on which Spiegelhalter has regularly appeared, has said of him: 'He is hugely loved by audiences because he is so obviously a searcher after the truth and no more or less. We love him because he's such a warm generous broadcaster – he is willing to engage with any question, however foolish, and he is humorous too.' He often features in our roundups on new studies that are statistics heavy, and we occasionally ask him to run 'introduction to stats' sessions for general news reporters and sub-editors, knowing that journalists will learn a lot while having a great time and never feeling patronised.

As a keen observer of daily science coverage, Professor Spiegelhalter one day tweeted about an inaccurate headline on drinking and pregnancy in the *Independent*. Jeremy Laurance, the newspaper's health editor, immediately contacted him by email offering to change the headline and inviting his input. I was copied into the exchange and what ensued was an almost comical laying bare of the differences between scientists and journalists. Spiegelhalter's proposed headlines were technically accurate, but too long and laboured. Laurance's edited versions were all compelling and pithy, but fell short of Spiegelhalter's exacting request for accuracy on a complicated finding. Laurance summed up the exchange aptly: 'This, David, is why I would make a terrible scientist and you would make a terrible journalist.'

Even if scientists don't always have time for journalists, you might assume that a respect for journalists would be a prerequisite for any press officer. Yet I remain amazed at just how many of them regard journalists with suspicion, even hostility. I remember at the height of the furore over the safety of the MMR vaccine in 2003, the BBC's Pallab Ghosh remarked to me that he sometimes felt that the Department of Health press office was trying to avoid the media altogether. The next day, I met with one of the department's battle-scarred press officers who said his team had given up on getting a fair hearing on MMR, and had resorted to putting BBC interview requests in a separate email folder which they never opened. I have met PR people whose contempt for journalists is visceral and who view my faith in them as naive. One head of comms at an arm's-length government agency told me that 'my problem' is trusting any of them. I certainly couldn't do my job without understanding that there are risks when engaging with journalists. But if you want to communicate your message to the wider public, you need to get to know journalists, work closely with them, find out what they need to do their job well, and offer it. How can you do that if you see engagement with journalists as the top item on your corporate 'risk register'?

I also happen to like and admire journalists. Much to my parents' chagrin, I turned down the offer of a place to study politics at the University of Leeds with its lovely campus accommodation to go to a bedsit in London because I wanted to study journalism. The Polytechnic of Central London (now University of Westminster) course was famously taught by working journalists, and two-thirds of my year group were mature students, several of whom were already journalists. Being surrounded by great journalists for three years led me to conclude that I wasn't good enough to be one. It did, however, confirm that I wanted to spend my career working with them. I have maintained that respect for thirty years and, I hope, imbued my colleagues with some of it. Of course, not all journalists are the same – as with politicians, scientists and press officers, there are good ones, bad ones, and atrocious ones. But one thing I tell academics frequently with real conviction is that you do not become a journalist on a national newspaper without being very, very smart.

Sometimes, of course, the communications officers who are hungry to work with journalists are curtailed by an overly cautious institutional culture, and it's heart-breaking to see fantastic science press officers ending up in organisations that just don't want to do media work. In the middle of a media storm about glyphosate in weedkillers, I called my friend Shira Tabachnikoff, who was then working for the European Food Safety Authority (EFSA) in a senior comms role. Both she and I had hoped that she could persuade the organisation to adopt a more open and proactive media strategy, but it was becoming clear that it viewed the media as a huge threat to be treated with maximum caution. EFSA had conducted all the rigorous safety testing of glyphosate and employed the experts that the SMC and media desperately needed to challenge grossly exaggerated claims about the cancer risk. Frustrated by what I saw as an overly uptight approach, I called to lobby her. She sounded miserable and explained that despite her best efforts they would not be putting anyone up for interview. In exasperation I asked her, 'What do people at EFSA do for fun?' For a terrible moment, I thought she was crying. Then I realised she was in the grip of a giggling fit. After what seemed an age of laughing, she eventually got the words out: 'Fiona, no one, absolutely no one, in EFSA is having any fun!'

It would be wrong, of course, to suggest that we never have run-ins of our own with journalists. There will be days when one or another of us is in despair, usually when some ridiculous non-peer-reviewed conference abstract with no available data has been covered prominently by all the newspapers, despite us sending out multiple comments from scientists saying the media shouldn't touch it with a barge pole. Or sometimes it is a day when we make a friendly request for a small change in a news report, and the journalist responds as if we are acting like Malcolm Tucker from *The Thick of It*.

Our most public row with the press was with the *Daily Express* back in March 2009. It's hard to imagine now but, at the time, there were multiple myths and inaccuracies circulating about the dangerous health effects of energy-saving light bulbs, and the *Daily Mail* and *Express* were both actively campaigning against their use. My colleague Tom Sheldon assembled a panel of experts to ensure the science journalists could sort fact from fiction. The next day, the *Express*'s front-page 'splash' was from our briefing. Under the headline 'Dangers of low energy light bulbs' it proclaimed:

> Serious concerns were raised yesterday about the toxic effects of energy saving light bulbs ... Doctors say scores of people are coming forward with skin complaints after

being exposed to the ultra-violet light emitted by the new-style bulbs. And the mercury powder inside them makes handling a broken bulb extremely dangerous. Exposure to high levels of mercury can cause itching, burning, skin inflammation, kidney problems and insomnia.

The other journalists in the room had written accurate stories, and Mike Swain, the science and environment editor at the *Daily Mirror*, wrote to us saying he could not believe the *Express* story had come from the same briefing he'd attended. But despite the other good coverage, an SMC briefing had somehow generated exactly the kind of scare story it was set up to avoid. Worse still, we had to explain what had happened to those experts who had agreed to take part because we had told them it would produce more measured coverage. Over the next few days, the scientists from the panel helped us identify eight key inaccuracies in the article. We sent the list to the *Express* journalist who had written the piece, a generalist who had just moved from the showbiz beat and who did not usually cover health or science, and her editors.

We had worked ourselves up into such a ball of righteous indignation that our next step, in hindsight, was very misjudged. We forwarded the complaint to all the journalists on our lists, with a note saying that, in future, such briefings would not be open to non-science specialists. Before we knew it, the *Guardian* media supplement and *Press Gazette* were on the phone. Later that day, a *Guardian* story went up under the heading '*Daily Express* attacked by scientists' group over "inaccurate" light bulb story'. It detailed our complaint and a response from the *Express*'s news editor, Greg Swift, who said the paper stood by its story, describing it as 'a factual and accurate account of the SMC briefing'. He criticised our decision to send that email, claiming it contained 'inaccurate and damaging allegations' and that it was 'unfair to single out a journalist'.

In our fury, we had assumed that the regular science journalists from the *Express* would share our dismay at their paper's inaccurate report but, of course, they wanted to support their colleague who had been publicly humiliated. They announced that they would not be attending further SMC briefings. A few weeks later, a science organisation pulled out of one of our press briefings because they had heard about the boycott. The row was discussed at an SMC board meeting a few weeks later, and I talked about how we had inadvertently painted the *Express* into a corner. Kenny Campbell, then editor of the *Metro*, interrupted to say: 'No, Fiona; you painted yourselves into a corner.' It was a fair point. The SMC cannot operate unless we work *with* journalists. We learned some hard lessons during that incident, and over time we have been able to repair the relationship with the *Express*.

Occasionally, tensions arise over what journalists perceive as SMC bias. In 2013 when the government announced the new NHS data-sharing project, Care.Data – a way of allowing scientists to access anonymised GP patient records to do medical research – the initial public response was mostly negative. As a result, in early 2014 we were asked by the Wellcome Trust and the Medical Research Council to run a briefing on why sharing data was good for medical research, in preparation for the expected rollout that spring. We lined up four speakers: Professor Liam Smeeth from the London School of Hygiene & Tropical Medicine, Professor Peter Weissberg, medical director of the British Heart Foundation, Dr John Parkinson, director of the Clinical Practice Research Datalink, and Richard Stephens, a cancer patient. In the time it took to arrange the briefing, a media storm had broken out, with privacy campaigners and GPs objecting to the Care.Data scheme on the grounds of insufficient consent and because data could be shared with pharmaceutical and insurance companies who would profit from it. The speakers at the briefing made a compelling case for the research benefits that sharing data would make possible, but the journalists accused me of assembling a biased panel and demanded to know why we hadn't included experts who opposed the scheme. A *Guardian* journalist said he knew of scientists who opposed sharing data and promised to send me their names, and a *Mail* reporter suggested that the whole briefing smacked of a set-up by the Department of Health.

It was a bruising encounter, and one we have thought long and hard about. Ultimately, the SMC's job is to represent the main-stream view of the scientific community and convey that consensus to reporters, not to cover an issue from all sides. If there are oppos-ing views among scientists, we work to ensure they are reflected in our output but, in this case, there was a strong and long-held consensus in medical research circles about the benefits of sharing medical records with researchers. The journalists, however, were unimpressed.

There was a similar scene at a July 2014 press conference on statins, a commonly used group of medicines that can help lower cholesterol to reduce risk of heart attack and stroke. What journalist David Aaronovitch called the 'Statin Wars' kicked off that month when the National Institute for Health and Care Excellence changed the recommended threshold for people to begin taking statins: previously you had to have a ten-year risk of cardiovascular disease of 20 per cent but the new guidelines dropped that to 10 per cent, making an additional 4.5 million people eligible for treatment. The decision prompted an angry response from some high-profile doctors who saw it as yet another sign of over-medicalisation – the excessive use of drug treatments when lifestyle changes would deliver the same health benefits. The debate about over-medicalisation is a legitimate and important one, but campaigners often end up misleading the public about the dangers of certain medications. In this case, the overwhelming scientific evidence and consensus favoured the benefits of statins. But, fuelled by unsubstantiated claims and small or weak studies about the risks, the dispute raged on with minority dissenting views often being accorded equal space alongside the huge body of reliable scientific evidence. Even veteran medical journalists, such as Fergus Walsh from the BBC, admitted they were struggling to report the story with so many conflicting claims to consider. Experts at the British Heart Foundation and other medical research bodies, meanwhile, had begun to fear that, like the MMR furore, this could have a huge impact on public health.

We assembled a panel of six experts who had either conducted the trials themselves or whose work brought them into close contact with the research. One, Professor George Davey Smith, had been a sceptic about statins in the early 1990s, arguing that their use should not become widespread until they had been tested in randomised controlled trials, which began to appear from 1994. Since then, he had been involved in many studies of the available evidence, which had clearly demonstrated the safety and effectiveness of the drugs. All six professors gave details on the many large, multi-centre randomised controlled trials that had demonstrated that statins were both safe and effective.

As the briefing ended, Ben Spencer, the *Daily Mail*'s brilliant young medical correspondent, challenged me for having amassed a biased panel, claiming he could find six professors from other universities who would put the opposite case. If he was right, the SMC would indeed have been displaying bias. But I knew he wasn't. There were one or two cardiologists who campaigned against statins, and a lot of GPs who felt they were offered too freely, but I knew there was not a significant group of professors of cardiology who took that view. When it came out, Spencer's report was balanced and accurate, acknowledging the consensus and stating in the very first line: 'Six professors from British universities have dismissed fears about statins.' However, the row had been witnessed by the other journalists at the briefing and Nigel Hawkes, by that point writing for the *British Medical Journal*, included it in his story:

> Fiona Fox, Director of the SMC, defended her decision to invite only pro-statin experts to the briefing. The 'vast majority' of cardiac and statin experts believed that the evidence was overwhelming, she said, and it was not the centre's job to provide a platform to a minority who did not and thereby project a false image that the debate was equipoised when it was not.

I understand where these journalists are coming from. No one wants to feel as if they are being hauled in front of the scientific establishment to be given a party line. Scepticism and challenging authority are healthy instincts in a free press, and where government departments and scientists are saying the same things, journalists may understandably perceive a closing of ranks. That does not mean journalists are always right. In the end, we don't hold these press conferences to endear ourselves to journalists. Indeed, we proceed knowing full well they may cause tensions or irritate some in the room, but when it comes to claims about the dangers of life-saving drugs like statins, we want the public to understand where the weight of scientific evidence lies.

The trouble with including viewpoints from outliers or a small minority in science is that it can create 'false balance', where the public think that mainstream science is equally divided when in reality there is a strong scientific consensus on one side. This is a tricky thing to get right, and we have agonised over our role in this.

At our tenth anniversary event at the Science Museum in 2012, then ITV science editor and future member of the SMC's advisory committee Lawrence McGinty warned us to avoid silencing genuine, informed scientific 'mavericks'. He argued that it could backfire not just in terms of missing out on important advances in science, but also because dismissing lone voices could ultimately damage public trust in both the media and science more generally. 'I think we have to be careful that we're not seen as some kind of totalitarian or authoritarian conspiracy,' McGinty argued, adding: 'I think the way to do that is to occasionally give the mavericks a say.'

McGinty's words were a hit with journalists in the audience and became a talking point at the drinks party afterwards. He is of course right that the history of science has been punctuated by visionaries who questioned the status quo and were chastised by the science establishment before ultimately being proved right. But they are few and far between.

Pinning down the scientific consensus is not always as straightforward as it is on issues such as statins or climate change. On several subjects where mainstream science is divided, such as the relative harms of cannabis, the link between certain pesticides and bee decline, and whether cancer screening saves lives, the SMC has taken care to reflect the opposing views of scientists in our output. Nor does a strong consensus mean that a subject is definitively settled. Scientists exist to prove each other wrong: that is how we advance our collective knowledge. Dr Philip Campbell, former editor-in-chief of *Nature*, used to tell audiences that big journals like his would kill to publish the new study that overturned everything we thought we knew about climate change, provided it was top-class science. The excitement in our office was palpable when we thought there was a study proving the harmful effects of eating GM foods. But with that GM study, as with any other, extraordinary claims needed extraordinary evidence. The key to all this is the quality of science. In the end, if a maverick is right then he or she will prove that through publishing good-quality research. Then they are no longer labelled a maverick.

But for every maverick proved right, there are many more who confuse and mislead the public about where the best evidence lies or what it says. So when journalists and others challenge us on being biased, the answer is not to appease them by finding outliers who reject the mainstream view. I would much prefer to miss the occasional genuine maverick than for the SMC to be responsible for misleading the public on important health issues such as the safety of a vaccine.

That said, the SMC has always made the case for scientists to embrace debate rather than calling on news organisations to try to shut it down. Most of the vaccine experts we met in the early 2000s had devoted much of their recent time to publicly knocking down discredited researcher Andrew Wakefield's claims about a link between MMR and autism. It is interesting that they nonetheless did not back Matt Hancock in spring 2019 when he was looking into new laws to force social media companies to stop anti-vaxxer messages spreading online, and that they were also generally opposed to making vaccination compulsory for health workers. We tend to agree with these scientists that driving anti-science views underground rather than debating them openly simply fuels conspiracy theories, and risks making martyrs of people with fringe views.

I also feel it's not a good look for science to be making demands about who should be given a platform by the media. I once made the mistake of asking a friendly journalist over a boozy lunch to use a particular expert – who was regularly getting their facts wrong – a little less often. He replied that, since I had asked him to use that particular expert less, he would make a point of using them more. Frustrating at the time, but an important lesson for me.

Clearly, there are still problems in the way that the media covers science. But overall, I am in the glass-half-full brigade. The UK media has a huge appetite for science stories and still invests in specialist science reporters. In some countries, science, health and environment reporters are more of an endangered species. Here in the UK, by comparison, science reporting is in rude health.

People are often surprised that I am so upbeat about the state of science journalism, given our remit and my criticism of some aspects of science reporting. But for every example of poor report-ing, there are hundreds of news pieces that convey important and complex science to a mass audience every day, from the *Today* programme to the *Sun*. Anyone who simply sits back and shakes their head at the daily failings of news reporters is missing the chance to make it even better. At the SMC, we have amassed many concrete examples of media coverage that has been improved and enhanced by the active involvement of good scientists. Things are not always perfect, and we are entitled to complain when a jour-nalist gets it wrong, but we mustn't forget to celebrate each time it's right. And every day, I see plenty worth celebrating.

10

A DYING BREED?

In defence of the science press officer

I DON'T CONSIDER MYSELF a proper science press officer. My background is in PR, not science, and even now I struggle to read some scientific papers. I have never had to write a press release about research, and still marvel at those who do. But science press officers are most definitely my tribe. I arrived at the SMC from a sector where it was natural to catastrophise for effect – whether aid agency or lobby group, a bit of exaggeration was justified as part of a broader attempt to raise funds and awareness.

In science, it was different. After years of idealising journalists, I had entered a world where scientists and their press officers saw themselves as purveyors of truth and accuracy. In my past jobs, hyping a story a little to get a slot on the ten o'clock news would win plaudits. In science, this approach was frowned upon. I liked my new world. Most of the science press officers I encountered had a science background rather than a PR one. Many studied science to degree or PhD level, but were not sure the 'bench' was for them. Others had worked as lab scientists but wanted a change. For them, a career as a science press officer offered the chance to stick with the science they loved. As a 'type', they tend to care passionately about how science is reported. But I think this type of science press officer is becoming an endangered species, and I want to lead the conservation campaign.

To understand anything about science in the media, you really need to know what science press officers do – more so since some estimates claim that PR professionals now outnumber journalists by six to one. Some describe the process of getting scientific findings into the public domain as a kind of pipeline or conveyer belt. At one end are the researchers, who may have laboured on their research for years before finally having the findings accepted by a peer-reviewed journal. Next come the science press officers from, variously, the university, institute, funder or publisher, who translate those findings into a press release, or sometimes several press releases, for a more general audience. Finally come the journalists, who use the press releases as part of their work in writing an account of the science for their audiences, adding their own spin and interpretation. I don't know precisely what percentage of science stories you read every day come from press releases, but I'd be willing to hazard a guess that most science and health reporting is shaped in some way by science press officers. John von Radowitz, science correspondent at the Press Association for over thirty years, said on his retirement that he and his colleagues could not have done their job without science press officers.

During my obsessive following of the Leveson Inquiry into journalistic standards (see Chapter 9), I watched Paul Dacre, then editor of the *Daily Mail* and known to some as Britain's 'scaremonger-in-chief', give his evidence in full. Dacre was loved and loathed in equal measure, but even his enemies acknowledged that he was a brilliant newspaperman who knew exactly what his 'Middle England' readers wanted. Lord Justice Leveson raised the issue of health coverage and questioned him about a *Mail* news story that had sensationalised a study on a new cancer risk, headlined 'Cancer danger of that night-time trip to the toilet'. My delight quickly turned to mortification when Dacre reached into his file and produced the university's press release on the study, then proceeded to quote from it: 'Just one pulse of artificial light at night disrupts circadian cell division ... damage to cell division is characteristic of cancer.' Ouch! Obviously it was pretty galling that the editor of the *Daily Mail* was shifting the blame for scare stories to a science press release when we know the news media are pretty adept at over-egging health scares or cures without any outside help. But the exchange did highlight a real issue in science media relations.

There are reasons why some press officers have a rather more relaxed attitude to accuracy than others. Some, like me, have come from outside science and are used to crafting press releases to get noticed. To this group, deliberately playing down a press release seems counter-intuitive, even negligent. Others may be under pressure from their university or institution to get namechecks and a higher profile as a means of attracting students and funding. Some feel it's not their place to challenge eminent senior academics about whether they are over-claiming for their work. Others try but fail. Whatever the reasons, the SMC decided early on that we couldn't advocate for more accurate and measured science journalism if we didn't also promote these values in science media relations. Our goal was not just to get scientists doing more media work, but to support them doing so in a way that helped drive up the standards of science reporting.

This occasionally landed me in hot water with science press officers. One clash I remember was when I went public about an egregious example of a hyped press release. It was just days after I had given my own evidence to the Leveson Inquiry, and I was conscious that I had used my limited time there to focus exclusively on the problems with journalism. A science journalist from the *Sun* called to alert us to a press release about a new study investigating whether silver compounds can be toxic to cancer cells. As often happens, the journalist was sceptical about the release and was asking for expert comment to help him convince his editor to spike it. Under the heading 'A silver bullet to beat cancer?', the top line of the press release read: 'Lab tests have shown that silver is as effective as the leading chemotherapy drug – and may have fewer side-effects.' Far from including any caveats or cautionary notes, the press office even included a note in the email claiming that the study confirmed the quack claim that silver has cancer-killing properties.

It was already fairly late in the day and the story was for immediate release, which in itself is bad practice for a press release from a peer-reviewed publication. We managed to get a comment from Professor Edzard Ernst, a German scientist who has spent his career specialising in the study, and evidence-based criticism of, 'alternative medicine'. We sent it out to our lists immediately. It read:

> This is an interesting test-tube experiment demonstrating that various forms of silver can kill cancer cells. While this line of enquiry is certainly worth further study, it would be very premature to draw any conclusion in terms of the treatment of human cancer. A plethora of compounds have similar activity but, for a range of reasons, cannot be used clinically. Any recommendation to use silver in any shape or form to cure cancer patients would, at this stage, be wholly irresponsible.

Several journalists got back to say they had convinced their editors not to touch the story. But others ran with it: the *Daily Mirror* had the headline 'Silver safer than chemotherapy and just as effective', while the *Daily Mail* ran it under 'Silver bullet for cancer: metal can kill some tumours better than chemotherapy with fewer side effects'.

I didn't mince my words when writing about the story later:

> I think anything that appears to offer patients real hope
> of cures and treatments for killer diseases should ring
> massive alarm bells and be handled with special care. If
> newspapers and press officers could follow the credo that
> you need extraordinary evidence to make extraordinary
> claims we would lose much poor science coverage over-
> night. I'm not sure we need a Leveson for PR, but I do
> think if we are asking newspapers to clean up their act
> and stop over-claiming for small provisional studies, we
> should do the same.

It wasn't just the press office in question that was upset with me.
There was some understandable resentment among press officers
in general that we were being sanctimonious about science press
releases without acknowledging the luxury of our position. After
all, we are gloriously free from many of the pressures that university press officers are under. We don't have pompous senior
scientists refusing to let us moderate their claims, or corporate
marketing managers breathing down our necks to get more name
checks. We don't even have to write press releases. But it is precisely because of our freedom from these institutional pressures
that we are well placed to voice these concerns. Indeed, I've often
raised them at the behest of science press officers who feel they
need to be said but are unable to do so themselves.

Nor is it just press officers who have highlighted this problem.
I first heard about Dr Chris Chambers and Dr Petroc Sumner in
2011. These two psychology researchers from Cardiff University
had found themselves caught up in a media storm when their
research was widely quoted in coverage of that summer's UK
riots. Their study had found that people whose prefrontal cortices

contain lower levels of GABA, an inhibitory neurotransmitter, also tend to have an impulsive personality. The study and the university's press release made no mention of rioting, but PA reported their findings under the headline: 'Brain chemical lack "spurs rioting"'. That piece was in turn picked up by the *Daily Mail* with the headline 'Rioters have "lower levels" of brain chemical that keeps impulsive behaviour under control', while the *Sun* heralded a 'Nose spray to stop drunks and brawls'. The hyperbolic headlines snowballed, and soon Chambers and Sumner found their research cited in news stories and blogs across the world. Horrified by the experience, the duo decided to take on the media.

Their intervention was popular with some scientists and bloggers. But I was wary. These scientists, who had no background in journalism or media relations, were now being given a platform to pronounce on how to deal with bad science reporting. At a panel debate in the Royal Institution in March 2012, they offered a plan for a 'kitemark' that would adorn every science story in the newspapers to 'enable readers to distinguish the type of journalism that everyone admires from churnalism and science fiction'. In a *Guardian* article from October that year, they called for journalists to routinely check their pieces with scientists, a suggestion that flies in the face of journalistic best practice whereby subjects are not able to see and approve a story in advance. Characteristically they made an intelligent and compelling case for science to be treated differently from other subjects, but their naivety was clear. The piece finished with the lines: 'No doubt some journalists will object to our arguments because we are intruding upon their professional sphere. This is true – we are intruding. But to those who object, we would ask, what is your primary motivation? Is it simply to produce a story with an angle or is to communicate science accurately and accessibly?' Every journalist I know would answer that question one way – their primary motivation, indeed their job, is to produce good stories with an angle.

I may have had my reservations about the approach of these two scientists but I admired their ambition and energy, and of course, I shared their goal. (They are also fantastic company at parties, a highly prized quality at the SMC.) I was on that 2012 panel debate too and since meeting them then, we have enjoyed a blossoming collaboration, with Chambers joining our board for some years and Sumner working closely with us on various research projects. The more they worked on the quality of science journalism, the more they directed their attention away from the reporting to an earlier stage in the communication process. Like others before them, they started to realise that some of what they were criticising in terms of poor reporting had originated in press releases. They were learning the hard way that it is not in the scientific community's gift to change the news media. As Chambers said, 'We've got zero chance of changing newsroom culture (my earlier escapades in this area taught me that). But we can change what happens in the universities because we basically ARE the universities.'

Being scientists, they decided to design a study to test the extent to which exaggerations emerged in press releases. They set out to identify the source of distortions, exaggerations or changes to the main conclusions drawn from research that could potentially influence a reader's health-related behaviour. It was a retrospective quantitative content analysis, which means they attempted to identify consistencies by systematically coding and identifying themes or patterns. They examined 462 press releases on biomedical and health-related science issued by twenty leading UK universities in 2011, alongside their associated peer-reviewed research papers and news stories.

I was on the advisory committee for the research project and was proud to be associated with it. But not everyone in science communication was so positive about what was being proposed. Some had fair criticisms of the study design. It had been a challenging study to set up and the authors were the first to acknowledge its limitations. Others saw the very proposal of the study as an unreasonable attack on a group of press officers trying to do their best in difficult circumstances. Around the time the two researchers were recruiting universities to take part in the trial, I had been invited to speak about the SMC's work at a Russell Group heads of communications group. I arrived early and sat through a discussion about the proposed study led by people who clearly did not know about my involvement. Some were supportive, but others were hostile and to my dismay a couple even reported on their attempts to stop their university taking part. One described it as an 'insult'. I was gobsmacked. These comms professionals represented the UK's top research universities but were objecting to their own activities being researched. It was also my first introduction to the type of senior comms directors now frequently being hired at universities, who are tasked first and foremost with protecting the brand and the reputation of a university. Fortunately, thanks to some heroic efforts from science press officers themselves and the persuasive skills of Chambers and Sumner, the authors eventually got the buy-in they needed, and the trial went ahead.

The study found evidence that when there was exaggeration in news coverage, it was often also found in the press release. The authors argued that improving the accuracy of academic press releases could therefore represent a key opportunity for reducing misleading health-related news. When the findings were published in the *British Medical Journal* (*BMJ*), I ran my own intensive PR campaign to ensure that vice-chancellors and other senior academics were aware of and discussing the findings. I urged science press officers to embrace the findings and understand the influence and power they held in shaping how new research was reported and ultimately understood by the wider public. This was no time to get side-tracked by defensiveness or a circular discussion over who was more to blame. As science press officers, it seemed imperative that we should welcome good-quality research that could help us improve the status quo. I also felt that some press officers were trying to have it both ways. Many of those who were sensitive about the *BMJ* study were the ones who complained that they were not respected or valued in their organisations. Yet here was a group of scientists who considered press officers so important to the process of science reporting that their contribution needed to be studied.

One of the practical measures we developed to improve standards in science media relations was a new labelling system for press releases, introduced in autumn 2018. The idea came from an important and influential report, 'Enhancing the use of scientific evidence to judge the potential benefits and harms of medicines', published by the Academy of Medical Sciences (AMS) in June 2017. I am a huge fan of the AMS, led for many years by the inspiring Dr Helen Munn. The report had been a response to a request from Professor Dame Sally Davies, the chief medical officer for England, to do something to help the public to work out where the best evidence lies on drugs like statins, hormone replacement therapy or Tamiflu – where conflicting advice is circulating. The press team at the AMS commissioned a poll for the media launch of the report, which revealed that when it comes to making decisions about whether to take a medicine, only 37 per cent of the public trust evidence from medical research, compared to 65 per cent who trust the experiences of their friends and family. Those figures spoke to the fears that prompted the research in the first place. As a nation, we invest millions of pounds and employ medical researchers to rigorously test what works, only for people to give equal or greater weight to something they see on social media or from a relative.

How to improve this ratio is what I think we now call a 'wicked' problem. Easy to identify; less easy to fix. One of the many things I love about the AMS is the way it does its reports. Not for them a hurriedly prepared document launched with great fanfare only to be left on the proverbial shelf. It tends to work on its reports for about two years and gets advance agreement from key players in the medical research community that they will lead on any specific recommendations that the report makes.

Along with other media bodies, we were approached to take on several of the proposed recommendations. One of these was the idea of a traffic light system for press releases. The intention was to signal at a glance whether new findings were at an early stage and therefore not yet very reliable, or whether they came from large clinical trials involving hundreds of humans and therefore could be deemed more solid. The project was something of a poisoned chalice: the idea that press officers would slap a red light on their own press release, signalling to journalists that they shouldn't touch it with a barge pole, was never going to work. Similar concepts had been explored previously and never got anywhere. But the AMS was persuasive, and we thought such a system might work as a potential de-hyping device to 'nudge' scientists, press officers and journalists in the right direction at a time when there were plenty of other things nudging them the opposite way.

As it turned out, we quickly ditched the traffic lights. Instead we worked with scientists, press officers and journalists to come up with three labels for use at the top of each press release on new medical research findings. The first would state whether the research had been peer-reviewed, indicating what stage of completion it was at. A second label would show the type of study – whether it was a systematic review, randomised controlled trial, observational study, literature review, case study or opinion piece.

A third label would aim to highlight whether the study had been undertaken in humans, animals, human embryos or cells.

A few press officers viewed the labelling system, like the research on press releases, as some sort of thinly veiled attack on their integrity. One was fond of reminding us that the SMC had ourselves run press briefings where scientists had exaggerated their findings. Entirely true, but not a good reason not to introduce a labelling system. Mostly, however, the system was welcomed, not as a kitemark to judge whether a particular study was 'good' or 'bad', but rather as a way to show journalists at a glance the kind of research it was and what stage it was at.

After a successful pilot, where ten press offices reported that they had found the labels easy to use and a useful reminder to check they had put all this information into the press release, we introduced the system to science and health journalists. Most stressed that they already checked for these things in press releases, but agreed it might be helpful to have that label at the top to help them make an even quicker assessment about whether to cover a story: a significant benefit to time-strapped journalists who might be faced daily with hundreds of press releases. Most also said they could see themselves showing the labels to over-eager news desks as a way of knocking down potential stories they felt weren't newsworthy. Job done.

The final step was recruiting senior scientists, vice-chancellors and institute directors to champion the labelling system. I don't imagine such eminent people have huge amounts of time to devote to thinking about the quality of their organisation's press releases, though on the rare occasions I have raised this with vice-chancellors with a scientific background, they have been enthusiastic. But the ultra-competitive environment they now have to operate in means that they are under multiple pressures. For many universities, student recruitment ends up subsidising research, so it makes sense to prioritise attracting new students. Professor Paul Boyle from the University of Leicester was a great champion for the scheme, having previously led Universities UK's work on research integrity. As he told *Times Higher Education*:

> We all know how – particularly in medical literature – one day a glass of wine is a good thing for you, the next day it's not, and there are many examples of that. With this in mind it's important to come up with a simple system that will help journalists understand what they're dealing with when a story comes to them.

This wasn't about pointing the finger at anyone involved in the communication of science, he said. Instead, it was a response to ongoing debates about good practice in research and how best to evaluate that.

Today, over forty-five universities, research institutes and publishers proudly display the labels, including the *Lancet* and the *BMJ*. Several other countries have expressed interest in following Britain's lead and the US-based EurekAlert, the biggest and most important science press release agency internationally, has acknowledged the system as the inspiration for a similar 'tagging' process for all press releases posted on their site.

Labelling press releases is a small and modest change but, for me, its significance lies in what it shows us about science press officers. It's hard to think of any other branch of PR that would consider smacking a label on the top of a press release to tell journalists why they should *not* plaster its contents on the front page. But science press officers are a special breed.

Let me give you one real example of that special breed: Dr Barnaby Smith was in charge of media relations at the Centre for Ecology and Hydrology (CEH) for thirteen years. The centre is a world-class research organisation focusing on land and fresh-water ecosystems and their interaction with the atmosphere. Smith had been a scientist at CEH before moving into media and communications. When he first came to see me in 2005, I was wary. Scientists didn't always make great press officers. But Smith proved me wrong within weeks.

He knew all the scientists in his research institute and could explain their research and its implications. He was proactive. Whenever a story touching on the centre's work hit the head-lines, Smith sent us a list of scientists available to comment with detailed information about their areas of expertise. He was on my speed dial, and that of every UK science and environment journal-ist, and would quite often answer my calls from an experimental field trial where he was already with the very experts the media needed. This responsiveness meant CEH scientists have featured heavily in TV news over the years. When I ran an emergency press briefing on the 2015/16 winter floods with four experts from CEH, the then director of communications at the Met Office called me, furious that they had not been involved and demanding to know how this had happened. The explanation was simple. When we sent multiple emails over the Christmas holidays to every scientist and press officer with expertise in flooding, Smith responded every time. One of those emails asked whether anyone thought it would be feasible to run an emergency press briefing on the floods on the first day back after Christmas. No one else replied. But Smith thought it was important and, a few days later, we had four CEH experts in our office along with seventeen national news reporters keen to hear from them.

Barnaby Smith is the type of science press officer that I worry we are losing: a press officer who loves scientists and science, and cares about how it's presented to the public; who wants to help answer journalists' questions; who believes that experts should be part of the national discussion; and who wants to make the best scientists available to the public at times of crisis or when science is contested. There are still some Barnaby Smiths around – but not as many as there used to be. And worryingly, when they leave their jobs, they are often replaced by people with a different skill set. I would love to see an analysis of the changes to job titles and job descriptions in the field of press and PR over the past decade. When a press officer moves on, the ad for their post tends to list a much wider set of required comms skills, and often barely mentions working with news journalists. One science press officer we hadn't heard from for a while told us her job title had changed to 'senior communications business partner' and told that a big part of her role now involves 'change management'.

It's important to state here that I am still struggling to understand the changes I have observed; the factors involved are often complex and opaque. They also vary among sectors. Changes in university media teams differ in interesting ways from those in research institutes, funding bodies and so on. Occasionally, an organisation will announce a new strategy and explicitly tell us that things in its media team will be changing and why. But mostly we are left wondering why science press officers we used to speak to daily have fallen off our radar. I never doubt that they are working incredibly hard and being pulled in many directions. I know comms officers who have had to support the bereaved parents of a student who died by suicide, who have gone door-to-door in student halls to hand out leaflets during a meningitis outbreak, and who have manned a GM garden display at the Chelsea Flower Show. They do not have the luxury we have of a clear focus on science in the news. As part of our twentieth anniversary plans for 2022, we have commissioned Helen Jamison, a seasoned science communicator and former SMC staff member, to do a report on the changing role of science press officers to ensure that the SMC and the sector has a more in-depth and rigorous understanding of the trends that will shape science PR in coming years.

In the meantime, it is with some trepidation and in a spirit of humility that I try to characterise these changes here. I am open to the possibility that I have misunderstood them, but I think an honest assessment of these changes is required to assess whether or not the UK research community is losing something of value to the public. By way of kicking off that discussion, I suggest that there are three main factors involved here: the changing media landscape; the changing nature of universities; and the professionalisation of science communications.

The biggest change facing all press officers in recent years is the opening up of the media landscape to such an extent that it has become possible to bypass the 'traditional' media completely. Before the arrival of the internet, the main way to get our stories and key messages out there was through the mass media. Now we have multiple ways of communicating with target audiences. Importantly, these new channels are often popular with scientists and science press officers, allowing them to control the way stories get out rather than having to cope with pesky journalists oversimplifying the science, insisting on 'balancing' it with critics or adding their own spin. Many senior comms people talk enthusiastically about moving away from an outdated 'media first' approach, and critically many scientists like the control they have over this content and don't miss the days of seeing their research 'dumbed down' in the mainstream news. Job titles have changed from 'press officer' to the more generic 'media manager' or 'comms manager'. And these staff are as likely to be writing blogs, making videos or curating content for in-house websites as they are speaking to journalists. A whole new skill set is required for these media managers, including digital comms, content management, social media and internal communications. I talk regularly to science media officers who admit that dealing with journalists and getting science stories into the media is an ever-diminishing part of their job. When the media and communications teams of all seven research councils were merged into one UK Research and Innovation communications team in 2019, it became a team of a hundred, only nine of whom were allocated to media relations. I see more and more organisations signalling that they don't see relations with the media as a major part of their future communications.

Running parallel with the changes in the media landscape has been the radical transformation of UK universities. Tony Blair's goal of getting 50 per cent of young people into higher education was first achieved in 2017, but the ongoing evolution of universities away from public utilities towards corporate enterprises was well under way before then. Higher numbers of students and far more substantial annual fees have seen universities forced to operate more like businesses, with students now often referred to as customers. One consequence of these huge changes is that research communications staff now tend to make up a small team within a huge marketing or fundraising department. One press officer at Rothamsted Research moved her family from Hertfordshire to Liverpool to take a job working with the pro-vice-chancellor for research and impact at the University of Liverpool. But soon after arriving, she found herself working instead as part of a much larger team and being asked to demonstrate that her comms aided marketing and recruitment. Like so many whose first love is science communication she decided to move on. Of course, it makes perfect sense to employ limited resources according to the needs of a university and to recognise that universities have a broad range of audiences including students, funders and government. But it's also true that the public interest in hearing from scientists may no longer be a top priority for a university comms team for whom the wider public is not a key target audience.

I recently spent months attempting to get an introductory meeting with a new head of communications at a top research-led university. Like most people at that senior level, her predecessor spent much of her time dealing with reputational issues such as social inclusion and funding, but she was very supportive of her research media team, and we were in regular contact. When I eventually met the new head, she was perfectly friendly but indicated that media was not a priority. She explained that in her view the media work 'tends to do itself' and said she had been recruited from government for her change management skills; the main challenge for her comms team was to anticipate changes and put PR plans in place to limit any fallout. Visiting another university, I discovered that the entire research communications team had imploded. The popular head of media, an ex-journalist with a passion for the university's research, had been moved sideways after an external review suggested there was too much focus on news and not enough on marketing and brand management. His two science press officers promptly resigned. I met with the new head who had come from a commercial background and spent the entire meeting telling me how irritating she found academics.

As with all my observations, there are just as many exceptions. Many universities, including UCL, Edinburgh, Warwick and Reading, have fiercely protected press officers specialising in science and news. On a recent trip to the University of York, I was taken to five departments including psychology and AI. Samantha Martin, the university's deputy head of media relations, used the walks between faculty buildings to fill me in on everything about the scientists I was meeting. Each researcher talked to me about previous media work: what had gone well, and what hadn't. Their enthusiasm for engagement with the press – and, by extension, the public – was inspiring, as was the warmth they showed for their press officer. By the end of the day, I was exhausted but exhilarated. Not only by the amazing scientists I had met and the long list of briefing ideas I was leaving with, but also because it was exciting to see that being a senior press officer at a research-intensive university could still be the incredible job I had discovered when I first arrived in science. When I asked Martin and her colleagues why York had bucked the trend I was seeing elsewhere, she said it was down to the director of external relations, Joan Concannon, who believed that media was still an important part of their job. I am grateful for her and others like her, but I believe this issue is too important to be left to individual champions. Nor is it enough to simply hope that the pendulum will eventually swing back in the other direction, given time.

While media teams in universities have changed a lot, other scientific bodies have retained a strong focus on science and the media. The four national academies of science, medicine, engineering and social science all have strong media teams, as do research organisations such as the Francis Crick Institute and the Institute of Cancer Research. Perhaps because of their close relationship with the public, patient-research charities including Cancer Research UK, the British Heart Foundation and Alzheimer's Research UK maintain strong media teams, as do the big journals such as *Nature*, *Science*, the *BMJ* and the *Lancet*.

The third factor driving change is what I call the professionalisation or corporatisation of science communication. In many ways, this is a consequence of the positive culture change I have charted in this book. Organisations that just two decades ago might have had one or two former scientists doing the odd bit of media work now have teams of professional communicators who are expected to bring a much more sophisticated and strategic approach to their role. Rather than being media-driven and reacting to events, scientific bodies ask what they are trying to communicate, to whom and for what purpose, and use the answers to set strategic objectives and priorities. Craig Brierley, head of research communications at the University of Cambridge, explained to a meeting of Stempra, the science press officers network, how his team wants to focus its limited resources on 'game changing research at the university', rather than in responding to every one-off media enquiry. He pointed to examples such as Professor Magdalena Zernicka-Goetz, whose research on early embryonic cells has prompted a broader global debate within science about whether the internationally recognised fourteen-day limit on embryo research should be changed.

A press officer at a plant science institute described how a huge part of her job has now become the management of a global scientific meeting, after an external strategy review established that this was the best way to achieve its goal of raising the institute's profile with scientists internationally. The Wellcome Trust, meanwhile, has recently launched a new strategy prioritising mental health, infectious diseases and global warming, and made it clear that its media relations and communications activities will focus on these. Such clarity is impressive. Here is the institutional goal, and here is the communications strategy to deliver it. But more broadly, of course, this kind of strategic communication and prioritisation means something else has to give, and we often find what gives is the responsive media work and the agility to drop everything when a science story breaks. In other words, they're not performing the very basic press office function of helping journalists to reach experts and get answers to their questions.

Critics may say I'm just one of those over-fifties who cannot accept that the 'legacy' media is dying. I understand that perspective, and there may be some truth in it. But the SMC is constantly monitoring and adapting to the dramatic changes in the news landscape. And, as things stand, the media is still a massively important part of our national life. It continues to set the agenda and influence public opinion. Print newspapers may be dying, but millions of us are reading their same news content online and it is often driving social media content. My twenty-one-year-old son has never read a newspaper and rarely watches TV news. But the stories he sees on social media are routinely links from mainstream, reputable news outlets. And there is some evidence that people are returning to trusted news outlets, especially during a crisis such as Covid. The Reuters Institute of Journalism Digital News Reports for 2020 and 2021 both documented an upsurge in people using traditional news media, particularly the BBC.

Mainstream news media still reaches and influences the general public, not just the 'science-curious' group that many media officers are now creating content for. If you care about public attitudes to issues such as vaccines, climate change or pollution, then you have to focus at least some of your efforts on news.

Taken collectively, these three broad changes raise a key question. If we accept that the news media remains one of the most important ways to reach the 'general public', which press officers should now answer the questions posed by journalists about science? Covid has put this question centre stage. Journalists and the public needed answers from scientists more than ever during the pandemic, yet science press officers who had worked with us and with science journalists in previous crises were no longer as available to contribute because their focus was now elsewhere. There were several university media teams that we did not speak to once throughout the two years of the pandemic.

In April 2021, I was invited to speak at a special event to mark the first anniversary of Oxford's Covid vaccine project. Speaking alongside vaccine co-creator Professor Sarah Gilbert and the head of the Oxford Vaccine Group Professor Andrew Pollard, as well as government scientists Sir Patrick Vallance and Professor Chris Whitty, who were all there to pay tribute to the scientists responsible for this remarkable achievement, I wanted to praise Oxford's media team for recognising the importance of supporting its scientists in talking to journalists and answering their questions.

In her opening remarks that day, Professor Louise Richardson, Oxford's vice-chancellor, said that Covid has shown the public that universities are not only places where students are taught but also where life-saving vaccines are developed and therapeutic drugs tested. She added that the high media profile of such scientific achievements would attract the brightest students and best researchers to the university.

We all benefit from scientific research, whether we know it or not. But in today's world it is not enough to simply do that research and leave it there: we also need to explain it clearly and accessibly. Good science communication can bridge the gap between what scientists do, and how and why that matters to the rest of us. It can foster meaningful discussions that build greater understanding and support for scientific research, improve public health and inspire new generations of scientists. My hope is to persuade Britain's universities and research institutes that, amid the important corporate, reputational, strategic and marketing messages, there should always be space for the communication of science to the media.

11

FOLLOW THE SCIENCE

The challenges of reporting on and in a global pandemic

COVID-19 IS THE FIRST STORY I have been involved in that was, for many months, the only story in the news. It took up the entire running order of the main TV news bulletins and was reported on by every available journalist in the newsroom. It was the only story in twenty years that all five SMC press officers worked on simultaneously and around the clock. It was also a huge test of how media and science work together. As the country plummeted into lockdown in early 2020, communicating the science involved became a delicate balancing act between government messaging, scientific research and accurate, measured reporting. The shared sense that 'we are all in this together' applied to scientists, journalists and communications officers – all trying to provide the public with clear, authoritative information. But shared goals do not always equate to a shared approach, and once again we found ourselves grappling with that age-old dichotomy: the desire for simple, clear 'messaging' versus the messy, complex, preliminary and uncertain picture that actually represented the science.

It was in early January 2020 that the SMC team began to notice a few stories about a mysterious new virus written by foreign correspondents in the international pages of the press. There was nothing to suggest to us at that stage it would arrive in the UK. But it was added to the 'watch list' of topics in our daily media monitoring. As the weeks progressed, though, it became clear that human-to-human transmission was happening, and media interest started to build. When a mother and son who had been in Wuhan in China tested positive in York, the story was taken on by the health and science journalists and it moved firmly to the front half of the newspapers.

As there had been no reported deaths in the UK, those early tabloid headlines like 'UK on killer virus alert' convinced some that we were simply in the grips of classic media fearmongering. This was the sort of thing the SMC was set up to counter, but we soon started to grasp that this was not a typical scare story. In February, I pointed out in my blog that there was a difference between alarm and alarmism, noting: 'The SMC is in close contact with many of the top scientists working on this virus, including virologists, epidemiologists, immunologists, public health experts and global health researchers. All of them are worried.'

I felt as if everything the SMC had ever done had been a dress rehearsal for this story. For decades, infectious disease experts had been warning of the dangers of such a crisis. Now it had arrived, and my team was as ready as it could be. We had a database of 3,000 leading scientists, many of whom we had worked with on previous outbreaks, including MERS, Zika and Ebola, and all were prepared to speak to a news-hungry media around the clock – quite literally. For a long time the SMC team was as busy at 10 p.m. as at 10 a.m.

In our line of work, one of the most striking things about the Covid crisis has been the degree to which top scientists were willing to do media work. We had been involved with plenty of stories where they had shied away, including Climategate and Charlie Gard, but things felt different with Covid. For eighteen months you could hardly turn on the TV or radio without encountering a scientist commenting on the pandemic. And not just on the 'posh' channels such as Radio 4, so loved by academics – *Good Morning Britain*, *The Jeremy Vine Show* and LBC talk shows all regularly featured scientists. The scientific community seemed to realise that building the public's understanding of the virus and trust in science would be critical to tackling the crisis. To those who ask me what good science communication looks like: this was it.

Our first press briefing was on 22 January 2020, with a panel of UK experts explaining what little we knew at that point. It was so packed that Tom Whipple from *The Times* had to squeeze onto a window ledge. Over the following eighteen months we ran over two hundred press briefings for science and health reporters and issued over 1,500 roundups and rapid reactions, three times our average workload.

Many top independent scientists were recruited to produce data and analysis directly for the government. The speed with which this was achieved and its impact on the pandemic was amazing to witness, and there is no doubt that it saved lives. It was also very important for public trust to have scientists outside government gathering this data. But it presented a familiar dilemma for us: once again scientists were subject to the constraints of government communications and messaging. Normally the prospect of university scientists waiting for permission from Number 10 SPADs to announce their data would be absurd – but during the pandemic, they often felt they had to.

Another challenge for us was that governments generally view scientists disagreeing with each other in the media as unhelpful.

Tim Cowen was a senior comms expert brought into government early in the pandemic to help coordinate science communication across all departments. Each time we met, he would reflect on his colleagues' frustration at all these scientists out in the media delivering contradictory interpretations on everything from the effectiveness of face coverings to whether mass testing was useful. I understood the frustration, and I did write to all the scientists on our books urging them to be mindful of the impact of their statements on public behaviour. But I argued to Tim that it was neither possible nor desirable to have it any other way. Science does not lend itself to the clear single messaging that the government favours. It's messy and complex and preliminary and contradictory. More so when it's about a completely new virus that no one yet understands. There was no scientific consensus on Covid, as there is for example on climate change or MMR, because there simply wasn't enough data from which anyone could form definitive conclusions.

There is rarely only one correct answer or opinion in science; it is not a set of facts and certainties, but a method of understanding the world by generating hypotheses and designing experiments to test them. Science advances by examining alternative explanations and by abandoning superseded ones. Eventually, we may reach some form of accepted view – we know the Earth goes round the Sun, and basic physics tells us the planet is warming. But on something like Covid, we were in a fast-moving situation where a large amount of new knowledge was being generated in a ridiculously short time. Eighteen months into the pandemic, we were still unsure about how long vaccine immunity might last and experts were debating whether we would face further nasty variants or whether the virus would evolve from a dangerous pathogen into another common-cold coronavirus. Issuing simple single messages may have been important from day one for government but it was not good science communication.

In my view, the problem was not with experts talking openly about complex, contradictory and incomplete knowledge but with ministers and government communications experts expecting them to deliver 'messages' and speak with one voice. I wanted politicians to acknowledge that there is a difference between science on the one hand and government decisions and messaging on the other. The science could inform the policies but should not be twisted to 'align' with them. Ministers parroting 'we are following the science' sounded great in the early days and was meant to reassure the public, but it was misleading.

One of the things that happens in a crisis is that you get the chance to explain aspects of the scientific method that would never make the news in 'peacetime'. In the early days of the SMC, I was often lobbied by senior scientists to do something to help the media understand more about the way science works. It was a difficult ask. Under normal circumstances, no busy news journalist is going to turn up to a media 'teach-in' about the scientific method. But Covid provided a platform to do just that. In mid-May 2020, the government's decision to lift lockdown restrictions was proving contentious and Bill Hartnett, head of communications at the Royal Society, asked the SMC to run a briefing on what 'following the science' meant. He provided us with a panel consisting of the society's then president – Nobel Prize winner Venki Ramakrishnan – as well as TV physicist Brian Cox and Professor Dame Linda Partridge, vice-president and biological secretary of the society.

Amazingly, thirty-three journalists joined our virtual briefing, and it was covered by national news outlets including *MailOnline*. The *Guardian* quoted Ramakrishnan as saying: 'Scientists will have got things wrong, but the beauty of science is that as new evidence comes in, you change your understanding of it.' They all made the point, one way or the other, that with Covid there was no such thing as THE science. One BBC reporter texted me halfway through the briefing – 'Enjoying the TED Talk from Brian Cox on the scientific method' – and it was true. It was like a mini lecture on the way science works, and at any other time it would have been utterly useless for news journalists. But the next day's papers contained powerful statements about the nature of scientific enquiry, like this one from Cox: 'Certainty arrives, eventually, because of the embrace of doubt.'

Having said that, at times of national emergency, the government needs scientific advice to inform its decision making; that is the role of the Scientific Advisory Group for Emergencies (SAGE), chaired by the government chief scientific adviser (GCSA). In past crises, we had noticed that once a scientist joined SAGE, they often seemed to stop doing wider media work, sometimes because they assumed they had to choose between advising government and informing the public, but also because they were asked by the government not to do media or to sign non-disclosure agreements or the Official Secrets Act. We had argued against this process in the past (see Chapter 7), so when we received an email in mid-February 2020 from a civil servant at GO-Science letting us know that a SAGE was being set up on Covid, we replied to express our concern about this happening again at a time when the public desperately needed access our best experts. I made a heartfelt plea that scientists joining SAGE would still be able to talk to the media. The response came swiftly:

I would like to reassure you that we do not restrict independent experts contributing to a SAGE from talking about their work in public or contributing their expertise to the media.

This was music to my ears and an early sign that GCSA Sir Patrick Vallance was taking openness seriously. And this was how it eventually played out. A variety of SAGE members did media work throughout the crisis, stressing that they were speaking in a personal capacity. This level of media access to SAGE members was unprecedented – and in my view a cause for celebration.

But not everything about SAGE was quite so open at the start. The names of its members were not published for the first three months, while the minutes from its meetings took another month to be released, and journalists were not able to assess the evidence on which its advice was based because the SAGE papers were also not being published quickly enough. I never understood the rationale behind this lack of transparency on SAGE at the start of the pandemic. On 24 March 2020, the day after national lockdown was formally imposed, I wrote to Alex Aiken, head of communications for government, outlining my concerns that the lack of openness was allowing journalists to present the system as rather mysterious and problematic, and that demystifying the SAGE process would help journalists see clearly what was and wasn't going on and could enhance public trust in the way scientific advice is given to government.

Aiken replied to say that the decision not to publish was out of a 'duty of care' to the membership after Whitty and Vallance had faced threats and online abuse. Not for the first time, I felt that this line of argument was misplaced. Of course, no one wanted scientists to be harassed or attacked, but all the SAGE members I knew wanted their names to be in the public domain, including the government's chief advisers. Several, including Sir Jeremy Farrar, had outed themselves in the media. As I suggested to Aiken, a duty of care might equally mean protecting these scientists from coverage that depicted them as part of a slightly sinister secretive group.

Eventually, in early May 2020, the government did finally publish the membership of SAGE after the *Guardian* published a leaked copy of the names. It was a terrible look for the government, with a national newspaper and several organisations claiming credit for forcing its hand. But it was the right thing to do and the members I knew were pleased. Soon after, SAGE started publishing minutes of all meetings as well as the scientific data and analysis used to inform SAGE discussion. It also started regular off-the-record briefings with the science and health journalists, where its members would go through the SAGE papers released that day and answer any questions. And yet still critics were claiming that SAGE was a secretive group – it was incredibly frustrating. While it may not be perfect, the group was the envy of many scientists around the world whose system of scientific advice was much more opaque than in the UK. In July 2020, I wrote a Thunderer column for *The Times* where I argued that SAGE had been more open than in any previous emergency:

> We have seen unprecedented levels of media engagement from scientific advisers . . . There were the daily Downing Street press conferences, often with Sir Patrick Vallance and Chris Whitty, and if we were left wanting more, we could turn on the TV to catch them and other SAGE members being grilled by politicians on select committees. SAGE members such as Jeremy Farrar, Susan Michie, Neil Ferguson and John Edmunds have been all over the media.

But SAGE continued to attract criticism. One of the issues was that, while SAGE became one of the most high-profile bodies advising on the national response to the pandemic, neither the public nor the scientific community really understood its role. The scientists on it were frustrated that people often blamed SAGE for making certain decisions when the group's role was only ever to offer advice; the decisions are made by politicians. They also felt people did not understand that the main work of SAGE and its subgroups was to answer questions put to it by the government. One common criticism was that the group modelled the health effects of growing infections but not of the social and economic disruption of lockdown. That's because that's what they were asked to model.

This lack of understanding of the way SAGE operated had been on full display when it had transpired that Number 10 Chief of Staff Dominic Cummings had attended meetings. People immediately speculated wildly about his role there. When I called the SAGE members I knew, they either hadn't realised he was present or else felt it was useful having him there. Mostly, they were surprised at the apparent outrage that the government should send officials to observe a meeting of scientists whose role was to offer timely and coordinated scientific advice to decision makers. As one of them said to me: 'It's kind of the whole point, isn't it?' After that latest controversy I invited Vallance and the previous GCSA, Professor Sir Mark Walport, to speak at a press conference for science journalists about the way SAGE works. They replied within minutes, and two days later, forty-five journalists got the chance to ask everything they wanted to know about the process.

Nevertheless, some scientists grew so frustrated by what they saw as the secretive and politicised nature of SAGE that they established Independent SAGE, an advisory panel of twelve scientists chaired by Professor Sir David King, GCSA from 2000 to 2007. I have always admired King – he was one of those bold scientists who resisted being pushed around by government SPADs. And the idea of setting up a group of independent scientists free from the constraints of government to feed into the national debate seemed sensible – indeed, that was what the SMC was doing. But I felt it was a mistake to name the group 'Independent SAGE': it unhelpfully implied that the official SAGE was simply a mouthpiece for government. It was also confusing – I was often asked questions by journalists about SAGE statements that were actually from Independent SAGE. As time went on, I felt increasingly frustrated by the way some of their members moved beyond their area of expertise and adopted strident policy positions on issues where the science remained uncertain. Members of Independent SAGE had total freedom to speak publicly, but I felt they did not always use that voice to good effect.

One of the challenges for this particular SAGE was the length of time it existed. During crises like 2010's volcanic ash cloud and the Novichok poisoning scandal in 2018, the relevant SAGE had lasted only a few weeks or months, holding a handful of meetings. This one lasted over eighteen months and held over ninety meetings. As one beleaguered member said to me after a flurry of articles criticising the group: 'We are not a secret cabal of "Official Government Advisers" plotting policy. We are a bunch of university lecturers trying to help politicians get things less wrong, who spend half our time trying to find the unmute button on Zoom.'

Amid the tragedy, chaos and uncertainty that plagued so much of 2020, it was a huge privilege to host regular conferences and briefings for the scientists involved in the many trials and studies that were helping the country chart the growth of the pandemic, understand more about the way the virus operates and find the most effective treatments. From Oxford's amazing RECOVERY trial, testing which drugs could reduce death rates, to Imperial's REACT study, providing regular data on the number of infections, these events were hugely significant in getting their findings out into the media, and generally went extremely well. Of course, not all of them went to plan – there was a mortifying one in March

2020 that we'd organised with Vallance and Whitty that I'd agreed to live-stream. Naturally viewers were unaware of my life-long cough from cystic fibrosis and Twitter was on fire with people concerned that I was giving Covid to two of the most important people in the country. I even made it on to Entertainment Daily, prompting a rare message from my son: *Mum, you're toast!*

Occasionally briefings were gazumped by ministers who wanted shiny announcements to make at Downing Street press briefings or in broadcast interviews. I remember one briefing we had lined up for a Monday morning to tell science journalists about a new in-hospital trial called PHOSP-Covid, looking at the long-term health impacts for patients hospitalised with Covid, only to turn on *The Andrew Marr Show* the day before and hear Health Secretary Matt Hancock announce it. It was picked up by general reporters working that Sunday and, as a result, the coverage contained very little medical science. Why should that matter, you might ask? Well, when scientific announcements are made by politicians rather than scientists, it's less likely that science reporters can discuss the research in detail with the scientists or clinicians responsible for it, which then enables them to summarise it accurately and accessibly for the wider public. It may not be disastrous, but it's nevertheless frustrating – particularly during such a period of uncertainty – that ministers would do this with no thought to how this might affect coverage.

The scientists were also furious. They had put aside time in a horrendous schedule to prepare for a press conference so that science journalists were well briefed. This happened several times during the pandemic. It could easily have been avoided: we often ran press briefings for science journalists under an embargo to coincide with a ministerial announcement, to enable politicians to get what they wanted while ensuring specialist reporters had access to the researchers involved.

Another problem we faced was that ministers would occasionally announce significant developments without making the data available. In mid-December 2020, for example, Matt Hancock broke the news of a new variant of the virus, then known as the Kent variant, which was believed to be more transmissible and potentially more deadly. The news that things could get worse rather than better was another major blow. Yet for many hours journalists were scrambling about desperately trying to access the evidence. I did what I usually do in these circumstances, and wrote to everyone I knew inside Public Health England (PHE), the Department of Health and Social Care (DHSC) and SAGE to express my frustration and underline how important it was that every new development be accompanied by as much scientific context and expert comment as possible, especially when there are gaps in the emerging knowledge and the potential for public alarm and misunderstanding. I mostly never got replies to such missives. This time, a senior PHE comms officer merely said they were broadly happy with the way it had landed. It said a lot about our different perspectives. One BBC journalist meanwhile sent me an email saying: 'Today was one of the worst moments of science communication in the whole pandemic!'

Media attention cast a spotlight on certain areas of science as never before, including immunology and virology. But the one that seemed to be loved and loathed in equal measure was epidemiological modelling. 'All models are wrong, but some are useful' is a favourite saying among scientists. When it comes to a completely new and unknown virus, however, they are essential. As one epidemiologist said to me: 'What else are you going to do: guess?' There were moments when it felt as if it was open season on modellers such as Neil Ferguson, or 'Professor Lockdown' as he became known to critics. Models work on best estimates when accurate figures are not available, and so they naturally tend to provide quite a large range of possible outcomes, and scientists are usually quick to emphasise the uncertainties involved. Media headlines often zeroed in on one end of the extremes, and then later commentators compared that figure to the real-world outcome to show how wrong the models were. Some lambasted scientists for, as they saw it, exaggerating the number of cases and deaths to justify lockdown. But this is both a misplaced attack on their actual role – which was to explain to the best of their ability what the available evidence indicated – as well as a serious misunderstanding of how models work and how they are used to inform decision making.

SPI-M, for example, is the modelling sub-group of SAGE. It had its first meeting at the end of January 2020, before a single case of Covid had been confirmed in the UK, but these scientists were already being asked to project how the pandemic might unfold in order to inform policymakers' decisions. In early March 2020, based on their modelling, the consensus was that Covid was circulating widely in the UK, could cause substantial hospitalisations and up to half a million fatalities, and in the absence of drastic social distancing measures, the healthcare system would rapidly become overwhelmed. Although new studies and data have since emerged, this general consensus has not changed.

We ran press conferences on the latest modelling, several hosting Professor Graham Medley, a modeller from the London School of Hygiene & Tropical Medicine (LSHTM) and co-chair of SPI-M, who would brief science journalists on the modelling used to inform key government decisions about newly announced changes to restrictions. Sometimes we tried to improve the way models were covered by the press, including running an event with Professor Azra Ghani from Imperial and Dr Adam Kucharski of LSHTM to demystify the inner workings of epidemiology. We were ably helped by Professor Dame Angela McLean, co-chair of SPI-M, who sent us a checklist to share with journalists. Key points included: don't only report the biggest number you see; ask the modellers 'Which bit of this are you most uncertain about?'; and don't let scientists get away with point estimates – they should always report ranges.

At the end of the day, it's vital to remember that models are only projections and will rarely be 100 per cent accurate; they must be analysed and used with caution. As Professor Medley described them: 'Models are a tool, and a really good screwdriver makes a poor hammer, but can be used to open a can of paint if necessary.'

All the data thrown up by various models were just one small part of the challenge that became known as the 'infodemic' – the flood of new scientific data arriving at breakneck speed as scientists around the world threw themselves into researching all aspects of the virus and the disease. Some estimate that almost 125,000 new papers on Covid appeared during the first ten months of the pandemic alone, and one scientist claimed that studies that usually took a hundred days from submission to acceptance were taking six days. There was a phenomenal amount of information to be sifted through constantly.

Perhaps the most difficult challenge for the SMC was the widespread arrival of the 'preprint', the term used to describe early scientific findings being shared by the authors on open servers which are accessible by journalists. These are preliminary scientific papers, which have not yet been peer-reviewed to establish if they're sound enough to publish. Preprints have been around in physics for years, but had only just started to enter the world of medical and clinical research before the pandemic. In June 2019, the SMC had made itself unpopular in some circles by issuing guidelines urging scientists and press officers not to send out press releases on preprints. In their enthusiasm for the benefits of preprints for research, scientists sometimes failed to consider the impact they might have on the way science reaches the wider public. We were especially concerned about early research findings that had implications for public health being splashed all over the news when those findings might be proven wrong, or at least not be robust enough to be published in their current state. Preprints are certainly useful in enabling the scientific community to interrogate each other's findings at an early stage, but it's much better for the public if researchers wait until the science is 'ready' before releasing it to the news media.

Before the ink was dry on our guidelines, however, we were breaking them ourselves in the face of the onslaught of Covid preprints. Far from waiting until the claims were published, we were running SMC briefings on preprints as well as gathering third-party comments for immediate release. On a couple of occasions, we reached the farcical situation where we were running press briefings before the preprint had even appeared on the server – a kind of pre-preprint.

Many preprints were good quality, providing data that helped scientists to make quicker progress and allowing policymakers, the NHS and the public to better understand the virus in real time. The trouble is that not all of them are equal. Flaky preprints attracted global headlines that were then shared with millions via social media. Scientists with little or no expertise in viruses were 'pivoting' into new fields and posting preprints that were then savaged by experts. One Canadian study, suggesting an extremely high rate of heart inflammation after Covid vaccines, had to be retracted due to a major mathematical error – but not before it had spread like wildfire on anti-vaccination websites and social media channels.

Nevertheless, with millions dying around the world, getting findings into the public domain quickly was imperative for scientists researching critical questions about the way the virus was transmitted, how long immunity lasted and who was most at risk. Global health leaders had long argued that it is morally untenable to allow evidence that can help scientists better control new infectious diseases to languish in sluggish publication schedules in the middle of an outbreak. All kinds of rules were being ripped up for Covid, and rightly so. I believe we were right to adapt our guidelines for the extraordinary times in which we found ourselves – but it does not follow that it's right to continue doing so during 'peacetime'. There will always be a risk of inaccurate information reaching the public, and that risk is not worth taking if there isn't a crisis making speed essential. Doing media work at the preprint stage should remain the exception rather than the rule.

For many reasons, Covid has been a 'science story' unlike any other I have seen. But it has been particularly unique because the pandemic has had an impact on all aspects of life. That has raised interesting questions in terms of how it is covered and presented by the media. BBC science reporter Pallab Ghosh argued at a debate in September 2020 that it was an 'everything' story and needed all kinds of correspondents from science to education to transport to politics. While this was patently true, I still felt the balance was sometimes wrong. In many ways Brexit was also an everything story – primarily political but with an impact on every section of society, including science. Yet no one expected science journalists to lead on Brexit. Similarly, in my view, all roads in the Covid story led to the science, and I was frustrated that science and health coverage too often took second place to the political analysis.

In the early stages of the story, from January to March 2020, that was indeed the case. Shaun Lintern, health editor at the *Independent*, told the *Press Gazette* that he was enjoying a rare moment of being the most important correspondent in the newsroom. But the supremacy of the science journalists seemed to dip when the daily televised Downing Street press conferences began in mid-March. Convention dictates that it is the lobby correspondents who attend Downing Street press conferences – but really there are no conventions when it comes to something as unprecedented as a global pandemic. Ministers had senior scientists at every press briefing, so it seemed obvious to me that the science journalists should lead the coverage instead of the lobby correspondents.

Some science journalists did make it on to this list and the numbers grew as the pandemic went on. But many told me that they had to battle their editors to be put on the list. One compared his newspaper to a football team, writing: 'The political editor is a bit like Ronaldo – he gets to take the penalties. I may occasionally be allowed to take a corner.'

Announcements made at the briefings generally became the big story of the day, but the trouble with political journalists taking the lead is that those stories tend to end up with more of a political slant, while the science takes a backseat. It seemed that many of the questions were only being asked in order to skewer the politicians, particularly trying to catch them out whenever there was a change in policy, asking them how they could justify these U-turns.

'MAYBE BECAUSE THE EVIDENCE HAS CHANGED!' I would yell at the TV. In the face of an evolving pandemic we desperately *needed* our political leaders to change their minds as new scientific data became available. But that is not how political journalists are used to operating – particularly having just endured an exhausting three years covering the adversarial and polarised politics around Brexit, with its constant U-turns and backtracking that they very rightly had to call out. But scientific developments are not the same as political opportunism, and I think the health and science journalists would have been better placed to report on them. Many, such as Victoria Macdonald from Channel 4 news, had covered the beat for years. They had an understanding of previous infectious diseases such as swine flu and SARS; they knew which scientists to approach; which research institutes specialised in coronaviruses; and which data were good quality and important. This specialism is critical to well-informed and illuminating reporting – journalism that leaves the public better informed rather than confused or suspicious about changes in policy.

The ridiculous daily ritual of announcing Covid test numbers at the Downing Street press briefings in April 2020 was a classic example. It became a kind of theatre, with Matt Hancock pulling ever bigger numbers out of his hat to gasps from his audience who were then determined to poke holes in the figures. Meanwhile, scientists were explaining the bewildering complexity around testing to science journalists, including the variation between different kinds of tests, false positives and false negatives, sensitivity and specificity, and so on. If only effective testing for Covid had been as simple as a numbers game.

Even before Covid, many journalists were reflecting on whether the 'gotcha' journalism favoured by many lobby correspondents has contributed to a corroding of our national discourse. Far from prompting a more honest and accountable style of governing, it has led political leaders on all sides to hire an army of SPADs to coach them in how to avoid answering questions that could get them in trouble. Even John Humphrys and Jeremy Paxman, the big beasts of political interviewing, talk in their memoirs about being troubled by their own role in this. These issues prompted reflection from some of the more thoughtful editors during the pandemic. Fran Unsworth, head of news at the BBC, circulated a May 2020 piece I had written on whether Covid needs a different kind of journalism to her senior editors, saying it raised issues she had been grappling with, while Dorothy Byrne, editor-at-large at Channel 4 news, delivered a keynote lecture called 'What journalists can learn from their mistakes during the pandemic' to the Reuters Institute for the Study of Journalism at Oxford.

My antipathy to some of the political reporting was not helped by hearing that it was putting some scientists off doing media work. One sent me a heart-breaking email: 'To be honest I've had it with the press. I'm being hounded by people who want to talk to us and when I do say yes it's always just a political agenda to point fingers and say who did it wrong.'

The reporting that really stood out to me during Covid was what I sometimes call the 'explaining' science journalism. It was science reporting of the highest standard I have ever seen, produced day in and day out. Editors reported hundreds of thousands of hits on articles explaining the R number, the latest modelling and the science of variants. Media experts talked of people returning in droves to trusted news sources, and one editor at *The Times* told me that the company's engagement data showed that readers wanted serious, in-depth expert reporting and analysis that they could trust and couldn't get anywhere else. Or, as he summarised: 'They want Tom Whipple explaining at length precisely what the virus does to the body.'

I think the appetite for this kind of reporting also has lessons for the way scientists interact with the media. I know many people who think scientists should not be too precious about where the boundaries of their knowledge lie, and that researchers working on one aspect of Covid are likely to be able to answer more general questions about it; I disagree. The strength of having multiple voices in the media relies on those voices speaking with a great depth of expertise, or as we said it in emails to scientists, 'staying in their lane'. With a completely new virus that no one yet understood, the last thing we needed was lots of scientists commenting from general knowledge. Some scientists seemed to enjoy the media spotlight a little too much. Some became ardent campaigners for particular policies like face coverings, mass testing or childhood vaccination, when the evidence was often finely balanced and uncertain. On a panel discussing Covid and the media in the summer of 2020, I was asked for my take-home message to the scientists watching. My answer was: 'In a nation of armchair epidemiologists, do your own good science. Study other people's science. Assess the quality of the science as it emerges. Then explain the science to the rest of us.'

There were moments during the crisis when we were confronted with the thorny question of what makes something a science story. Was the news that Prime Minister Boris Johnson had been taken into hospital with Covid one for us? What about the news that Dominic Cummings had broken lockdown rules? There were no easy answers, but if science journalists were covering the stories and asking us for statements then we tended to gather comments. One such dilemma was the news that broke in the *Daily Telegraph* on 5 May 2020 that Professor Neil Ferguson, a key member of both SPI-M and SAGE, had broken lockdown rules by meeting up with his lover. Ferguson apologised immediately and resigned from SAGE. I understood people's frustration and the criticism of his actions, but I never enjoy public shaming, and this one felt close to home. I was also worried that we might lose one of the best modellers in the country at a critical point in the pandemic.

As the story broke in the early evening, we debated whether we needed to solicit reactions from scientists. In such instances we often ask, 'Does science have something to say about it?' We felt it probably did, but we were very conscious this was a story about an individual's private life. I hoped that his resignation and apology would mean it would just be a twenty-four-hour wonder, and we decided to wait for the next day's papers.

The decision was made for us at 6 a.m. the next day when I was woken by Tom Feilden from the *Today* programme, asking for a scientist to come on to discuss whether Ferguson's actions would undermine the integrity of the research he had been working on. I emailed everyone on our Covid list and, despite the ungodly hour, had multiple volunteers within minutes. First up was Professor Sir Robert Lechler, then president of the Academy of Medical Sciences, who was fired up by commentators overnight suggesting that the scientist's resignation cast doubt on the integrity of the models informing lockdown. He reminded the millions of listeners that Ferguson was just one of a large team at Imperial, and that the models informing the SAGE advice came from multiple groups. Asked about Ferguson's conduct, Lechler said that he did the right thing by falling on his sword so quickly.

Another individual who had a hard time in the media for a few weeks was Kate Bingham, the life sciences venture capitalist appointed by the prime minister to run the Vaccine Taskforce (VTF). Early media reports often presented her as part of the 'chumocracy', appointed by her old friend Boris Johnson and married to a Tory treasury minister. But when we started running media briefings with her, we found her to be extremely good at communicating complicated aspects of vaccine commissioning and delivery.

In November 2019, however, Bingham was caught up in a media scandal. The *Sunday Times* wrote a piece implying that rules had been broken in her appointment and that she had provided confidential information about vaccines at a private investors conference. She and the Department for Business, Energy & Industrial Strategy (BEIS) denied the allegations, describing them as inaccurate and irresponsible. None were ever proved but the rest of the media reported them with an unabashed glee for several weeks.

The accusation that caught my attention, and that of many journalists, was that Bingham had hired a 'boutique' PR firm for the taskforce, allegedly costing over £600,000, despite having access to the government communications machine. Many deemed this scandalous, with Labour leader Sir Keir Starmer saying that 'you cannot justify that sort of money being spent', and a succession of presenters demanding that ministers justify the expenditure. My initial response on hearing the story was that using independent press officers was further proof of Bingham's good sense and independent spirit. In fact, neither viewpoint was accurate: we were all rushing to judgement without stopping to check the facts. I later learned that much of the work the external agency was hired to do was on communications for the recruiting of volunteers for the various UK vaccine trials because the BEIS comms team had neither the skills nor the capacity to cover it.

The press officers at Admiral Associates, the PR agency in question, had both prior expertise in science communication and were independent from government. They wanted to make Bingham and the other taskforce members available to the media and public. It seemed odd to me that so many journalists who had criticised government press officers in the past were suddenly outraged by the use of independent communications officers, especially given how important the vaccine was. As I wrote for *PR Week* at the time, I have been arguing for years that it is always better for science communication to be led by scientists, science press officers and science journalists. Almost everyone acknowledged that a successful vaccine was the main escape route from the nightmare scenario of multiple lockdowns. It's hard to imagine a stronger case for getting the communications right.

Bingham stood down from her role in December 2020, insisting that she had only ever been given a six-month contract and was looking forward to going back to her day job. But she later spoke in interviews about how the media row had been a huge distraction, affecting the whole team when they had a critical role to fulfil. When the vaccines that she and the VTF had secured arrived, and the UK led the world in its successful rollout campaign, the media turned her from a villain to a national hero. Newspapers ran glorious profiles and editors fought to run exclusive interviews. Admiral Associates stood back when Bingham did and the media relations for the VTF went back into BEIS comms. The next two heads, Dr Clive Dix and Sir Richard Sykes, did barely any media work and we never ran another press briefing with the VTF.

The briefings we ran on vaccines were by far the most positive aspect of our work on Covid, although not always straightforward. In November 2020, we ran one with Professor Sarah Gilbert and her colleagues, the lead developers of the Oxford-AstraZeneca vaccine. It became something of a cause célèbre when she and her colleagues announced their findings from the third phase of the trials. Unlike the Pfizer and Moderna announcements, which had both given one simple efficacy number, the Oxford-AstraZeneca trial had delivered three: overall the vaccine was shown to be 70 per cent effective overall, rising to 90 per cent in the group that had received a half dose and then a standard dose, and falling to 62 per cent in the group that received two standard doses. The global media appetite for these results, and the fact that AstraZeneca's involvement made the results market-sensitive, meant that scientists had only seen the top-line results the day before. They tried their best to explain the slightly messy results to journalists, but the truth was they themselves didn't yet understand why a lower dose would be more effective. They repeatedly reminded journalists that the findings would be written up in a full scientific paper in a couple of weeks.

Tom Whipple of *The Times* later wrote an opinion piece under the headline 'Oxford muddled a good vaccine with bad PR'. Despite the headline, the article was largely complimentary about the vaccine, but I called Whipple to disagree with his point that what we needed in a pandemic was clarity. It's more important that we have honest acknowledgement that scientific findings can sometimes be complex and uncertain, and scientists don't magically have all the answers. The comparisons drawn between the different vaccines in terms of their media relations were also unhelpful: we were in danger of valuing style over substance, seduced by slick communication rather than science. Notably, the Oxford-AstraZeneca team was far more open with the media, doing press conferences every time there was any new development or data, while the PR for other vaccines was more restricted and controlled. The last lesson I wanted anyone to take from this, least of all science journalists, was that scientists should become more polished and slick.

Of course, the Oxford-AstraZeneca vaccine had more travails to come. While more and more real-world data showed the vaccine was effective against severe disease or hospitalisation, haematologists began to see a tiny group of patients who developed a rare type of blood clot soon after being vaccinated. Because cases were so rare, and also occurred in unvaccinated Covid patients, it was difficult to piece together what was happening. By Easter 2021, the Medicines and Healthcare products Regulatory Agency (MHRA) had confirmed that it was investigating whether the blood clots were linked to the Oxford-AstraZeneca vaccine.

All drugs have side effects, and when you give a new vaccine to millions of people, it's possible there will be some serious adverse events. When the vaccines had first arrived, we and many other science bodies were invited on to a Zoom call by BEIS. They asked what we could do to support positive messaging on vaccines. In response I asked how the government was planning to handle media interest in side effects, and suggested we needed to prepare the public for adverse events. As any fans of BBC mockumentary

W1A will appreciate, the chair of the call said, 'Yes, exactly, yes', before swiftly moving on. What government comms people never seemed to grasp was that no amount of 'positive comms' will guarantee public trust in a vaccine if you run for cover at the first hint of a side effect. While the overall proportion of cases was still tiny, the numbers were going up and the media interest was intense. But my conversations with the science journalists reassured me that they were acutely aware of their responsibility to report this in a way that was neither downplaying a real risk that the public needed to know about, nor exaggerating the dangers in a way that could put people off getting the vaccine altogether. As they repeatedly stated, the risks of getting blood clots and strokes were far higher from catching Covid than from being vaccinated.

Yet again, the independent scientists closest to the developing situation and most clued up about the data were being urged not to do media work by their government minders. As the story grew in the days before Easter, we found several leading haematologists who were involved in treating some of the affected patients and advising the MHRA and others on the condition. One by one though, they replied to say they had been asked not to speak to the media by various government agencies and their NHS Trusts. The only contribution we received from official sources was a holding statement.

At 7 a.m. on Easter Saturday, I wrote another missive to government comms teams, reminding them that holding statements do not stop journalists from reporting on a story, that they will simply look elsewhere for additional commentary instead, and that while it was understandable they didn't want their scientists to engage with the media until they had more information, it was incredibly frustrating that they would try to prevent independent scientists from speaking up as well. I pointed out that what they were mostly achieving was annoying the science and health journalists who were the best hope of measured coverage over the coming days. I received no reply.

Luckily for us all, the vacuum left by the MHRA and DHSC over the Easter weekend was filled by responsible reporting, although journalists had to turn to a variety of scientists who were not experts on the condition. Most of those scientists had to stick to making general points about the risk–benefit ratio. I had some sympathy for the government's concern that the public might be scared away from being vaccinated. But asking haematologists not to speak to the media, when they knew most about this side effect and were seeing it in their hospital wards, was not a trivial matter. The story was prominently covered, acknowledging a horrible side effect that had been linked to the vaccine while also making it clear that the numbers of cases suggested there might be a one in 250,000 chance of getting this rare blood clot after the vaccine, and a one in a million chance of dying from it. Journalists explained the science clearly, and went out of their way to demonstrate that the benefits of taking the vaccine massively outweighed the risks, especially for older people. The *Sun*, so often dismissed by academics as a sensationalist tabloid, ran a front page with the headline '0.000095 per cent – Tiny chance of a killer clot after AZ vaccine'.

Then in the summer of 2021, another vaccine story looked as though it might cause an uproar in the media as the government took a different view from that of its science advisers over the question of whether to vaccinate twelve- to fifteen-year-olds. Other countries such as Israel and the USA had already begun vaccinating children, and it became clear that UK ministers saw it as one way to reduce transmission before the arrival of winter and avoid reintroducing any restrictions, as well as hopefully keeping children in school during the autumn term. But the Joint Committee on Vaccination and Immunisations (JCVI), tasked with advising government on vaccine strategy, was cautious. Children tend not to suffer severe symptoms from Covid and many are asymptomatic, so the justification for vaccinating children is different from that for adults, where the need was much more clear-cut. Children can of course still contribute to the spread of the disease, so many public health experts favoured vaccinating children to drive down infections in adults as well as children. However, evidence had also started to emerge that the Pfizer vaccine was linked with myocarditis, a heart condition that can cause an abnormal heart rhythm. Reports from the USA suggested cardiologists were also worried about changes showing up on the scans of young people with vaccine-related myocarditis, which were adding to the concern within the JCVI. This adverse event is very rare and we know more people get myocarditis from having Covid than from the vaccine, but it did affect the risk–benefit ratio and it was the JCVI's job to assess that.

In early September 2021, I was told that the JCVI had just voted against recommending vaccinating all children for the time being, deciding that, according to the evidence, the benefits were too small. Whatever you think of that advice, and many scientists we knew disagreed with it, this was an independent scientific advisory committee working exactly as it should, basing its conclusions on careful assessment of the evidence and resisting any external pressure. But I was immediately concerned about how this decision would be communicated to the media and public – and what would happen if the government went against this advice.

That evening, I asked a science journalist what he thought would happen if, hypothetically, the JCVI ruled against vaccinating children and government went ahead and did it. His answer was exactly what I didn't want to hear. In his view, that could not happen without creating a 'furore': the government had claimed to have followed the science throughout the pandemic and could not now take a divergent view on an issue as sensitive as vaccinating children. I argued that it shouldn't be shocking that an independent group comes to a different conclusion from government: the JCVI had a specific remit, primarily looking at the risk–benefit ratio of vaccines to individuals, but there were other factors to consider, including transmission rates and the impact on children's education, and so it was perfectly reasonable for the government to make a different decision. The idea that the media might not take that into consideration and instead spin the decision in a way that could turn it into a major row was frustrating.

On 3 September, I advised the JCVI to arrange its own press conference as soon as possible to explain its recommendation. I underlined how important it was to explain its decision while also acknowledging that the government could quite reasonably come to a different conclusion, and I pointed out that allowing this to escalate into a row would have long-term consequences for the committee, for the government and, most importantly, for childhood vaccination.

Professor Wei Shen Lim, chair of the JCVI's Covid committee, replied straight away thanking me for my support and assuring me that they were already preparing for a news briefing. I breathed a sigh of relief as the press conference took place a couple of hours later. The professor explained the basis for the committee's recommendation not to vaccinate, and that they had suggested the government might want to seek the chief medical officers' views on the wider public health factors. Within days, the chief medical officers had reported their advice to vaccinate children and the government announced this would start within days.

Of course, some journalists talked up the 'row' and early editorials decried this 'mixed messaging', but most took on board the reasons for the different approaches given by the experts on all sides. Their reporting was considered and balanced. There is no doubt that the difference between the JCVI's advice and the government's approach made it harder for parents and children to decide on whether or not to opt for vaccination. But what was the alternative in the face of this difference of opinion? For the government to pressurise the JCVI to arrive at a different decision, or stop it briefing media about its advice? That would have done far more damage to public trust. People understood that this was a complex issue but importantly that there was no scandal here and I enjoyed watching vox pops with parents and children who had clearly understood the scientific explanations for the different approaches they had seen in the news. For me, the importance lay in the proof of principle. Independent scientists had communicated the reasons for their decision and government had explained why they decided not to follow it. In time we may gather additional evidence that will help us judge the arguments made by both sides, but for now what matters is that this difference of opinion was played out in the open.

With clear successes and failures in how Covid was reported in the media and hopefully with the worst of the pandemic now behind us, there are lessons to be learned. I live in hope that we will have a proper independent inquiry, one that examines thoroughly which systems worked well and which did not. We need a constructive investigation that shows us how we can apply those lessons to a future crisis. I would love to see new rules establishing the principle of a clear separation between government and science communications. But what would not be helpful is a media narrative I find particularly unappealing – that of hindsightism and playing the blame game.

There are very few people in political or media circles who can say hand on heart that they warned us about a coming pandemic. Many commentators claim that they would have taken us into lockdown earlier, despite the fact that they barely mentioned

Covid throughout January and February 2020. For a period of time during the early months of the pandemic, I signed off emails to colleagues, friends, and family with #HumilityNeeded. It is not a quality I am generally associated with, but I felt the need for it keenly when so many people seemed to have such confidence that if only *they* had been on SAGE or in government we would have got this right.

That is not to say of course that everything went well with the UK's response. There was a heck of a lot that the government got wrong. Professor Martin Hibberd from LSHTM was in Singapore when news of the virus first emerged, working with public health experts there in pandemic preparedness. He watched bewildered as the UK government failed to implement the preparedness plans he knew had been developed here – measures such as mass community testing and contact tracing – from the very start of the outbreak. Singapore had a very similar plan. 'But the difference is they actually implemented it,' Hibberd said.

***

In September 2000, a report was published by the Economic and Social Research Council called *Who's Misunderstanding Whom?* It was the result of a year-long exploration of the relationship between science and the media led by Professor Ian Hargreaves, then director of the Centre for Journalism Studies at Cardiff University. With chapter titles including 'Collision course' and 'Maps of misunderstanding', the report concluded:

> To the question of 'Who's misunderstanding whom?', we answer that all the players in this particular drama have too long a history of misunderstanding each other. Unless we can do better, we will weaken our ability to make wise judgements about science, undermining science

and our ability as a society to make progress. Nothing less
is at stake.

When the SMC was set up twenty years ago, I had a vision of what success for us might look like. I wanted a culture change so that senior scientists would come to view talking to the media as an integral part of what it means to be a scientist, while news editors would see science reporting as an area to be led by specialist science, health and environmental journalists. When I look at how scientists and the media have interacted throughout this awful pandemic, both those changes have largely come to pass. Much was – and remains – at stake for our society, but in the relationship between science and the media today I see cause for celebration and hope.

ACKNOWLEDGEMENTS

First and foremost, I need to acknowledge my colleagues past and present. They barely get a mention in the book, but have been with me every step of the way. My interview panel knew that they were taking a risk recruiting someone with nothing more than an O level in biology, and consequently Baroness Greenfield immediately handed me her latest protégé, a supersmart science graduate called Becky Morelle (now science editor of BBC News). From that day on I recruited similar types. None of them ever talked about PR, or 'messaging', or reputation management at interview – instead, they all talked about their passionate belief in the scientific process and their hopes for a career ensuring that the science in the news was accurate and measured. They are what makes the SMC such a trusted and respected science press office.

Becky's colleagues and successors are, in no particular order: Tom Sheldon, Fiona Lethbridge, Helen Jamison, Ed Sykes, Claire Bithell, Alice Kay, Selina Kermode, Freya Robb, Hannah Taylor Lewis, Andy Hawkes, Ellie Friend, Nancy Mendoza, Natasha Neill, Robin Bisson, Michael Walsh, Simon Levey, Sophia McCully, Becky Purvis, Lyndal Byford, Tony Lomax, Heather Morris, Mark Peplow, Will Greenacre, Jonathan Webb, Joseph Milton, Lara Muth and Adrian van Schalkwyk. Additional thanks to Tom, Fiona and Freya for, between them, reading drafts of the entire book at various stages and providing help, advice, support, and welcome feedback that I was on the right track!

One of these science graduates, however, gets an extra special acknowledgement. Alex Durk walked through the door for interview in July 2019 for a role providing support to the press team and the CEO. One bullet point had been added to the job description at the eleventh hour – to support the CEO in writing her book. Little did Alex know what a huge part of his job this would become. It turns out that writing a book was something of a challenge for a woman in her late fifties who can no longer remember anyone's name, is incapable of dealing with tracked changes, and thinks the 'cloud' is something you see in the sky. Alex made up for all these failings. He worked stupidly hard on this book and often had the worst bits to do. I don't just think it would be a less good book without him. I think there would be no book without him.

Secondly, I must thank those who helped me with aspects of the book – from fact-checking certain sections, to sanity checks on judgements, to just helping me to remember things from 10 or 20 years ago that are rather fuzzy. I tried to make a note of everyone who, despite being busy, kindly responded to my request for a favour, but apologies to anyone I have missed out. If the book is wrong in places, that is my failing. But if it's mostly a fair recollection of events and describes the science-y bits accurately, then that is absolutely down to these people, and I am so grateful to them. They include: on GM foods, Professor Chris Pollock, Professor Giles Oldroyd, Professor Joe Perry, Dr Jonathan Jones, Professor Mark Tester, Professor Maurice Moloney and Roger Highfield; on animal research, Ather Mirza, Professor Max Headley, Dr Paul Brooker, Val Summers and Wendy Jarrett; on ME/CFS, Professor Carmine Pariante, Carol Rubra, Ed Sykes and Sarah Boseley; on human-animal hybrids, Professor Robin Lovell-Badge; on the Nutt saga and government scientists, Professor David Nutt and Justin Everard; on Climategate, Sir Philip Campbell and Simon

Dunford; on Fukushima and breaking news, Adrian Bull and Dr Barnaby Smith; for the journalists chapter, Clive Cookson, Jeremy Laurance, Justin Webb, Roger Highfield, Tom Feilden and Tom Whipple; for the press officers chapter, Professor Chris Chambers, Professor Louise Richardson, Mark Sudbury, Professor Petroc Sumner and Professor Rasmus Nielsen; and on Covid-19, Professor Adam Finn, Professor Calum Semple, Professor Graham Medley, Jeremy Laurance, John Davidson, Professor John Edmunds, Dame Kate Bingham, Professor Sir Peter Horby and Professor Steven Riley.

I also want to acknowledge the hundreds of scientists who aren't named here but who have featured heavily in the story of the first 20 years of the SMC. My publisher convinced me to drop the multiple declarations of love that peppered the early drafts, but I hope that they will know who they are nonetheless. The SMC can only ever be as good as the scientists who agree to work with us and let us offer their time and expertise to the media. The media does science better when great scientists do media better, and I love those scientists who do that. This book is for them and about them, even if their names are not on the pages.

I'd like to thank Olivia Bays at Elliott & Thompson. If anyone outside science buys this book and enjoys it, it will be down to the huge amount of time Olivia invested in transforming it from a book aimed at my immediate science circle to one that a wider audience might enjoy. I didn't always make that easy for her, but she was right.

A big thanks also to the SMC's wonderful chair of trustees, Jonathan Baker. I first met Jonathan when he was running the BBC College of Journalism, which was all about maintaining the very best journalistic standards. We share a passion for that essential news value of impartiality, currently under threat. It was Jonathan who used an appraisal three years ago to tell me to stop just banging on about writing a book and actually get on and do it. He was the only non-SMC staffer to read the book before it went to print, so I will of course blame him if it all goes wrong. A mention also for the SMC's board members past and present. Many CEOs tell me they endure their board, but ours has always been packed with impressive people who are too busy being effective in their own organisations to meddle in operations. They have challenged us in all the right ways, and many of our decisions about direction and approach lead back to their insights and wise counsel.

Last but not least, I must acknowledge my family and friends. 'The Girls': Eileen, Janet, Jenny, Siobhan and Pauline – a group of challenging, opinionated, strident women who have been a constant presence for over 30 years and are one of the great pleasures of my life. On science, as on other subjects, they will never let me get away with defending a position without a bloody good argument to back it up. My husband Kevin – the obsessive Celtic fan and inspirational teacher who makes sure to keep my ego in check but who encouraged me to write this book. He is a true champion of the enlightenment values that unite us in our love of the scientific endeavour. My son Declan – a young man just starting out on his life. Whatever he does, my main wish is that he will eventually find the kind of fulfilment and sense of purpose I have been lucky enough to enjoy. And my wonderful sisters Claire and Gemma, who take such pride and pleasure in what I do. We sometimes reflect on what it was about our upbringing by Irish immigrants in an unremarkable bit of north Wales that gave us each the self-confidence to end up becoming leaders in our chosen fields. Maura and John Fox would be proud that I have published a book. They would also have loved the party celebrating its publication – another trait handed down to the Fox girls.

INDEX